# Enhancing Cancer Care
Complementary Therapy
and Support

# Enhancing
# Cancer Care
Complementary
Therapy and Support

Edited by

Jennifer Barraclough
Bach Foundation Registered Practitioner,
Auckland, New Zealand

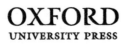

OXFORD
UNIVERSITY PRESS

# OXFORD
## UNIVERSITY PRESS

Great Clarendon Street, Oxford OX2 6DP

Oxford University Press is a department of the University of Oxford.
It furthers the University's objective of excellence in research, scholarship,
and education by publishing worldwide in

Oxford  New York

Auckland  Cape Town  Dar es Salaam  Hong Kong  Karachi
Kuala Lumpur  Madrid  Melbourne  Mexico City  Nairobi
New Delhi  Shanghai  Taipei  Toronto

With offices in

Argentina  Austria  Brazil  Chile  Czech Republic  France  Greece
Guatemala  Hungary  Italy  Japan  Poland  Portugal  Singapore
South Korea  Switzerland  Thailand  Turkey  Ukraine  Vietnam

Oxford is a registered trade mark of Oxford University Press
in the UK and in certain other countries

Published in the United States
by Oxford University Press Inc., New York

© Oxford University Press 2007

First published 2007
Reprinted 2008

Some subjects and themes in *Enhancing Cancer Care: complementary
therapy and support* have been previously discussed in *Integrated Cancer Care:
Holistic, Complementary and Creative Approaches* published by
Oxford University Press, ISBN - 13 978-0192630957, now out of print.

A catalogue record for this title is available from the British Library
Data available

Library of Congress Cataloging in Publication Data
Data available

Typeset by Cepha Imaging Private Ltd., Bangalore, India
Printed in Great Britain
on acid-free paper by
Biddles Ltd., King's Lynn

ISBN 978–0–19–929755–9 (Pbk.)

10 9 8 7 6 5 4 3 2

# Preface

Complementary and alternative, holistic, integrative, natural, unorthodox, mind–body–spirit are some of the many names given to a large and varied group of therapies that have become popular in cancer care. When delivered by skilled practitioners, and adapted to ensure their safety in any particular setting, such therapies can often help to relieve cancer-related symptoms and improve well-being and perhaps even to extend survival of people with cancer. However, deciding which approaches—if any—to choose in the individual case can be a daunting task. This book is a practical, evidence-based guide illustrated by clinical examples. It is written for both conventional healthcare professionals and complementary practitioners working in the fields of oncology, palliative care, or family medicine. It will also be useful for people with cancer who want to play an active, informed part in planning their treatment strategy.

Since the publication of my previous book on this topic, *Integrated Cancer Care*\*, this group of therapies has become far more widely accepted for use alongside conventional medical treatments. Even so, some mainstream healthcare professionals continue to be misinformed about these therapies or prejudiced against them, while some practitioners of alternative medicine remain suspicious and hostile towards orthodox medicine. Having spent many years working as a doctor in the UK National Health Service before embarking on a new career as a natural health practitioner, I can appreciate both perspectives but believe that the best way forward is through co-operation and mutual education, rather than competition.

Part 1 of this book presents the general principles of holistic cancer care, discusses the evaluation of therapies, and describes some different service delivery settings. Part 2 describes 16 specific interventions. Because no grouping of the therapies is entirely satisfactory, they are arranged in alphabetical order. I hope this compilation of chapters, all written by experts in the clinical and academic aspects of their chosen fields, will make a valuable contribution towards the care of people with cancer.

J.B.
*Auckland, NZ*

\* *Integrated Cancer Care: Holistic, Complementary, and Creative approaches*, edited by Jennifer Barraclough. Oxford University Press, 2001.

# Contents

# Contributors

**Jennifer Barraclough**
Formerly Director of Psycho-oncology,
Churchill Hospital, Oxford UK;
Currently Bach Foundation
Registered Practitioner,
Auckland, New Zealand

**Heather Boon**
Associate Professor of Pharmacy,
University of Toronto, Canada

**James Brennan**
Consultant Clinical Psychologist,
Bristol Haematology and
Oncology Centre;
Senior Clinical Lecturer, Bristol
Doctorate in Clinical Psychology,
Senior Lecturer in Palliative
Medicine,
University of Bristol, UK

**Elizabeth Butler**
Senior Nutritional Therapist,
Penny Brohn Cancer Care,
Bristol, UK

**Kerry S Courneya**
Professor and Canada Research
Chair in Physical Activity and
Cancer,
University of Alberta, Canada

**Alastair J Cunningham**
Ontario Cancer Institute and
Professor Emeritus,
University of Toronto, Canada

**Beverley de Valois**
Senior Lecturer,
Centre for Complementary
Healthcare and Integrated Medicine,
Thames Valley University;
Research Acupuncturist,
Lynda Jackson Macmillan Centre,
Mount Vernon Hospital,
Northwood, Middlesex, UK

**Claire VI Edmonds**
Research Associate,
Princess Margaret Hospital,
Toronto, Canada

**Tiffany D Floyd**
Assistant Professor,
Department of Psychology,
City University of New York;
Research Fellow,
Department of Psychiatry and
Behavioural Sciences,
Memorial Sloan-Kettering Cancer
Center,
New York, USA

**Bonnie Gabriel**
Registered and Certified Art
Therapist,
New Jersey, USA

**Nigel Hartley**
Director of Creative Living Centre,
St Christopher's Hospice,
London, UK

**Kara M Kelly**
Associate Professor of Clinical Pediatrics,
Division of Pediatric Oncology,
Columbia University Medical Center,
New York, USA

**David W Kissane**
Chairman of Department of Psychiatry and Behavioural Sciences,
Memorial Sloan-Kettering Cancer Center,
New York, USA

**Elena J Ladas**
Director of Integrative Therapies Program for Children with Cancer,
Columbia University,
New York, USA

**Joanne V Loewy**
Director, Louis Armstrong Center for Music and Medicine,
Beth Israel Medical Center,
New York;
Professor, Hahnemann Creative Arts Therapy Graduate Program,
Drexel University, Philadelphia, USA

**Barbara Lubrano di Ciccone**
Instructor of Psychiatry,
Department of Psychiatry and Behavioural Sciences,
Memorial Sloan-Kettering Cancer Center,
New York, USA

**Paola Luzzatto**
Registered Art Therapist (UK and USA),
Member of the Board of Directors for Art Therapy Italiana Training School,
Bologna and Florence, Italy

**Peter A Mackereth**
Clinical Lead in Complementary Therapies,
Christie Hospital, Manchester, UK

**Margaret L McNeely**
Physical Therapist,
PhD Student in Physical Activity and Cancer,
University of Alberta, Canada

**Sara R Miller**
Specialist in Integrative Medicine,
Penny Brohn Cancer Care,
Bristol, UK

**Diane O'Connell**
Principal of College of Healing,
Malvern, UK

**Clive S O'Hara**
Consultant Reflexologist,
Manchester, UK

**Doreen Oneschuk**
Associate Professor in Palliative Medicine,
University of Alberta, Canada

**Karen Pilkington**
Project Manager and Senior Research Fellow,
School of Integrated Health,
University of Westminster, UK

**Janet Richardson**
Reader in Nursing and Health Studies,
University of Plymouth, UK

**Ruth Sewell**
Lecturer in Integrated Cancer Care and Spirituality and Psychotherapist,
formerly at
Penny Brohn Cancer Care,
Bristol, UK

**Donald M Sharp**
Senior Lecturer in Behavioural
Oncology,
Oncology Health Centres and
Institute of Rehabilitation,
University of Hull, UK

**Jacqui Stringer**
Clinical Lead in Complementary
Therapies,
Christie Hospital, Manchester, UK

**Elizabeth A Thompson**
Consultant Homeopathic Physician,
Honorary Senior Lecturer in
Palliative Medicine,
Bristol, UK

**Andrew A Walker**
Clinical Trials Manager,
Oncology Health Centres and
Institute of Rehabilitation,
University of Hull, UK

**Leslie G Walker**
Director,
Oncology Health Centres and
Institute of Rehabilitation;
Professor of Cancer Rehabilitation,

Hull and East Yorkshire Hospitals
NHS Trust
and University of Hull, UK

**Mary B Walker**
Senior Clinical and Research Nurse
Specialist (Behavioural Oncology),
and Research Fellow,
Oncology Research Centres,
Hull and East Yorkshire Hospitals
NHS Trust
and University of Hull, UK

**Teresa E Young**
Research Co-ordinator,
Lynda Jackson Macmillan Centre,
Mount Vernon Cancer Centre,
Northwood, Middlesex, UK

**Jawaid Younus**
Medical Oncologist and Assistant
Professor,
University of Western Ontario,
Canada

**Catherine Zollman**
General Practitioner and GP
Educationalist,
Bristol, UK

## Chapter 1

# Introducing the holistic approach to cancer care

Jennifer Barraclough

## Summary

In many parts of the developed world today, patients with cancer have access not only to standard medical and surgical care but also to a wide range of other therapies that are grounded in a more 'holistic' philosophy of health and healing. Many such therapies have come to be regarded as valuable complements to orthodox medicine, but there is still scope for conflict due to differences in professional attitudes and beliefs. In this brief overview, the reasons for the increased acceptance and popularity of these therapies, the challenges of evaluating them in this era of evidence-based practice, and some aspects of service delivery are discussed.

## Introduction

Many of the therapies that used to be dismissed as 'quackery' or 'fringe medicine' are now recognized as having real benefits for patients with cancer. Their use alongside conventional treatments is being increasingly accepted, and often welcomed, by professionals in oncology and palliative care. While technical advances in surgery, radiotherapy, and chemotherapy continue to achieve greater number of cures and longer survival times, there has been a growing appreciation of the 'human aspects' of disease management—awareness that individuals are as important as their tumours, that the quality of life is as important as its length, that simple natural lifestyle measures sometimes help as much as sophisticated technology, and that the art of healing, the 'heart and soul' of medicine, will always have a place alongside the science.

The therapies described in this book are a diverse collection and in some ways they may appear to have little in common. Some are focused on the physical body, others on the mind or spirit. Some are grounded in conventional medical science, others in a different philosophy. Therefore, no generalizations about these therapies can be entirely valid, although they do share some important features, as discussed below.

Approaches include lifestyle modifications through diet and exercise; psychological and spiritual support for individuals and groups; creative expression through art and music; and a range of other therapies grouped under the umbrella term complementary and alternative medicine (CAM). The boundaries of CAM are flexible; it can be pragmatically defined as including any therapies that are not part of conventional Western medical training or practice. However, many such therapies now receive at least some coverage in undergraduate and postgraduate education programmes and are being absorbed into mainstream practice as evidence of their benefits builds up.

## Terminology

Some of the terms in this field are now used so loosely that they have become clichés. It may be useful to go back to their dictionary definitions.

*Complementary*: 'serving to fill out or complete', 'mutually supporting each others' lack', and 'combining in such a way as to form a complete whole, or to enhance or emphasize each others' qualities'. All the interventions described in this book can be complementary to the conventional methods used for the management of people with cancer.

*Alternative*: 'available as another possibility' or 'mutually exclusive'. Alternative therapies are used instead of conventional ones, not alongside them. The main focus of this book is on complementary rather than alternative usage.

*Integrated*: 'with various parts or aspects linked or co-ordinated'. Integrated (or integrative) medicine aims to combine the best of both complementary and orthodox care.

*Natural*: 'existing in or caused by nature; not made or caused by humankind'.

*Unorthodox*: 'contrary to what is usual, traditional, or accepted'.

*Holistic*: 'characterized by understanding the parts of something to be intimately interconnected and explicable only by reference to the whole'.

## The philosophy of holistic healthcare

What is now often called the 'holistic' model of healthcare has ancient origins. For example, in the fifth century BC, the Greek physician Hippocrates expressed some of its tenets when he said that the aims of medicine are 'to cure sometimes, to relieve often, and to comfort always' as well as 'to do no harm'; that 'it is more important to know what sort of person has a disease than to know what sort of disease a person has' and that 'natural forces within us are the true healers'.

Most of the key principles listed subsequently are perfectly in keeping with the conventional (orthodox, mainstream) approach of Western medicine, but some stand in contrast to it.

- An emphasis on the 'whole person' (body, emotions, mind, spirit, and social and physical environments). A harmonious inter-relationship among these different levels of the self correlates with good health. Conversely, disease states are linked with imbalance. Many of the therapies act predominantly on just one of the levels; therefore, it is often desirable to combine two or more approaches to cover all relevant aspects of a particular case. This contrasts with orthodox medicine, which has a narrower focus on diagnosis and symptoms and in which practitioners increasingly tend to specialize in one structural or functional part of the body

- Giving treatments that strengthen the innate potential for good health and resistance to disease, rather than those designed to suppress symptoms or directly eliminate pathology

- The use of natural modalities in preference to 'high-tech' interventions with chemicals, surgery, or radiation. However, terms such as 'natural' and 'organic' are vague and can readily be challenged. Natural treatments cannot be clearly distinguished from 'non-natural' ones, for example, many medical drugs are derived from plant or animal sources rather than synthetic chemicals. It is also important to remember that naturally occurring substances are not necessarily safe

- Encouraging 'self-responsibility' for health by marshalling the sick person's own sense of active involvement in healing. This calls for a collaborative client–therapist relationship, rather than the traditional doctor–patient interaction, which is more authoritarian. An illness may be viewed as a learning experience to draw attention to imbalance in the self and as an opportunity for personal growth; however, it is important that this concept of self-responsibility does not become equated with guilt about being ill

- Many, but not all, of the therapies are based on a belief that all things in the universe, although apparently separate, are manifestations of an energy that connects them all together. This ancient belief has recently gained support from studies in the 'new' schools of physics, biology, and psychology and has had some interesting consequences, for example, a closer dialogue between science and spirituality. According to the 'vibrational' model of the self, ill health is understood as an imbalance or weakening of the personal energy system. This contrasts with the orthodox medical approach, which is focused on the measurable material phenomena of anatomy, physiology, and biochemistry. Not everyone is open to theories about depletion of the vital force, imbalance of the personal energy field, or psychospiritual conflicts being important in illness. However, it is possible to benefit from the therapies without exploring their underlying philosophy.

## Why do patients use the therapies?

Surveys suggest that, in parts of the Western world, at least 50% of people with cancer are using one or more of the therapies, usually alongside conventional treatment, rather than instead of it. Patients who opt for this type of treatment approach tend to be younger, better educated, and more affluent than those who do not, and are more likely to be female. Some surveys have also reported higher levels of psychological disturbance and of dissatisfaction with conventional medical care. Wider use of the therapies has been encouraged through the growth of self-help groups, and of access to information through popular literature and the Internet—although the quality of such information sometimes leaves much to be desired. Hoped-for benefits may include:

- Relief from cancer-related symptoms
- Relief from side effects of conventional treatments
- Improved psychological adjustment and support
- A more active sense of choice and control
- A gentler, more natural alternative to conventional treatments
- Discovering a sense of meaning in the illness
- Remission or cure of the cancer

## Evaluation

Descriptive studies show high levels of patient satisfaction with the therapies, even when patients have opted to use them on the basis of personal interest and intuition rather than systematic research data. However, if the therapies are to be administered and funded on an equal footing with conventional treatments, more rigorous evaluation is required. Health services in most developed countries have been strongly influenced by the advent of evidence-based medicine (EBM) and the need for increasingly strict management of resources stretched by high-cost, high-tech treatments. Interventions are selected on the basis of proven clinical benefits and cost-effectiveness; their delivery must meet high standards of quality and their outcomes need to be audited. Quantifying change in physical symptoms is fairly straightforward, but devising valid assessments for the psychological, social, and spiritual spheres of life presents more of a challenge. While those working in the 'softer' specialities have recognized the need for EBM and made sterling efforts to meet its requirements, many would consider that some important aspects of the human condition are too intangible to capture using numerical outcome measures.

Therefore, there are differences of opinion regarding the most appropriate methodology that can be used to evaluate these therapies. Some argue that this should be exactly the same as that used in orthodox medicine. Others consider it essential to take into account the distinguishing features of practice in this field, for example:

- Treatment regimens are tailored to individual patient characteristics rather than standardized for a particular symptom or diagnosis
- Patients' own motivation and choice as regards type of therapy, therapist, and timing are important and this is denied to them if they are randomly allocated to a particular regimen
- The therapies are often used in combination rather than singly
- The timescale of response can be slow in some cases and there may be an aggravation of symptoms before improvement takes place
- Some of the desired outcomes, notably those in the psychospiritual sphere, are not easy to measure

Some regard the randomized, double-blind controlled trial (RCT) as the gold standard and the only valid means of assessing new treatments. Others argue that the RCT is something of a sacred cow and that qualitative methods are more appropriate in the field of CAM. Adapting delivery of a therapy to meet the design requirements of an RCT can turn it into a travesty of its original form.

Although there is a still a need for more well-designed research studies, there is now considerable evidence that the therapies can help to relieve cancer-related symptoms through specific effects, over and above the general benefits resulting from the additional time and attention given to each individual and from the surrounding mystique which may contribute to healing.

Most research to date has focused on quality of life rather than its length and oncologists are often reluctant to consider the possibility that some of the therapies might help to stem or even reverse the progression of cancer. There are many obstacles—scientific, practical, and ethical—to researching this aspect; yet for many patients it is of course of prime importance. Cases of 'remarkable recovery' following wholehearted commitment to the holistic healing approach are probably more common than is realized in conventional circles. The therapies have undoubtedly helped many others to achieve some kind of positive emotional and spiritual development, whether or not they survive their cancer.

## Professional attitudes

The 'orthodox' and 'holistic' camps are much more friendly and open towards one another than used to be the case. However, traces of the former antagonism and misunderstanding still remain, with extreme viewpoints represented on both sides.

Many professionals in oncology, especially nurses, are keen to learn more about CAM. Others, especially of an older generation, adopt a tolerant stance but do not really take it seriously. A die-hard minority—mostly doctors—remain highly sceptical and antagonistic. They go to great lengths to find flaws in research studies reporting that some of the therapies actually work. They dismiss any apparent benefit as a placebo effect—failing to consider that if a placebo can activate the patient's own powers of recovery, it could be the best medicine of all. Their scepticism is understandable with respect to those therapies that are claimed to act at a metaphysical level and do not seem to have any rational, scientific basis. However, until quite recently, even such common-sense natural interventions as eating more vegetables and taking more exercise were sadly neglected in oncology research. This is partly because more funds are available for pharmaceutical studies but it probably has something to do with professional attitudes as well.

Extremists on the opposing side believe that conventional oncology with its 'war against cancer' is on the wrong track altogether. They claim that the 'slash, burn, and poison' method of attacking the disease, combined with the overuse of 'suppressive' drugs to control the symptoms, kill more patients than they cure and can never produce true healing. Instead, they advocate natural methods of prevention and management. They may dismiss the great hard-won achievements of medicine and surgery in one fell swoop without offering any sound evidence to support their own claims. Again, this is a minority viewpoint and most complementary practitioners would agree that conventional medicine is essential in certain situations even if they believe it to be overused.

## Unwanted effects and limitations

The therapies are generally both safer and cheaper than conventional treatments. Many of them, such as aromatherapy and music therapy, are also a great deal more pleasant to receive. But some can have adverse effects, especially in the hands of unskilled practitioners. For example, herbal medicines can be toxic either in their own right or when they interact with orthodox drugs; there are occasional reports of infection or tissue damage with acupuncture and massage; and the various psychological approaches may worsen emotional distress.

Perhaps the most common criticism regarding the therapies is that they do not work and therefore lead patients to harbour 'false hopes', waste their time and money, and sometimes decline conventional treatments that would have been effective. In fact, there is considerable evidence to show that the therapies are beneficial when properly used but they cannot work miracles or provide an easy 'quick-fix'. Many of them require sustained patience and commitment from both client and practitioner.

There are few legal restrictions covering practice of most of the therapies in most parts of the world, although moves towards stricter regulation are currently underway in some countries. At present, the field is wide open to misguided or unscrupulous practitioners, which occasionally leads to tragedy. More commonly, the problem is that therapies are administered by personnel with sound intentions but inadequate training. This can include oncology staff, for a background in conventional medicine or nursing does not qualify anyone to practice CAM safely and effectively. Patients themselves can easily access literature regarding the therapies and buy 'natural medicines' over the Internet or from health food shops. All this amateur practice probably does more good than harm and with many of the therapies, self-help is perfectly acceptable and even to be encouraged. However, it can lead to indiscriminate and damaging overuse, through extreme diets, for example. It may also lead to the methods being dismissed without a fair trial. For example, the fact that an 'over the counter' homeopathic mixture has not helped does not mean that an individualized remedy, selected by a qualified homeopath after a detailed interview, would not be worth trying.

## Service delivery trends

Until recently, many of the therapies were only available in the private sector. Even now, those patients who can afford to do so may still prefer to go to independent practitioners who have no connection with oncology services. This gives them choice and control as regards which therapies they use and when, and enables them to be treated in a congenial environment without the distressing associations of a hospital or palliative care unit. All these are valid reasons for wanting to keep the therapies separate. It is also true that people value what they pay for.

Private therapy can, however, have disadvantages apart from its cost. Patients may not have the knowledge to choose the most appropriate therapy or therapist. If the therapy takes place without the knowledge of oncology staff, there may be unfortunate results, for example, unrecognized interactions between a 'natural remedy' and a medically prescribed drug. It is also likely to promote mistrust and misunderstanding. Instances of herbal or homeopathic remedies being secretly smuggled into hospitals or alternative practitioners advising patients to abandon their orthodox treatment are still reported. Such problems are less common now that complementary therapies are available alongside orthodox ones in many cancer treatment settings—a development that is being encouraged by many official bodies in the UK, USA, and elsewhere. This move towards integration is partly the result of patients themselves having become much more willing and able to challenge the authority and infallibility of orthodox medicine and to explore a wider range of approaches.

It may also be linked to other trends within cancer care during recent decades. One of these is the expansion of the palliative care movement, which is no longer confined to providing hospices for patients with terminal cancer but has expanded to cover the needs of patients in community and general hospital settings and some of those at earlier stages of their 'cancer journey' or suffering from other types of progressive disease. The palliative care approach has always emphasized the control of pain and other physical symptoms, included families and carers as well as patients, and taken a 'whole-person' perspective that includes the spiritual aspects of illness and dying. Another trend has been the emergence of psycho-oncology as a subspecialty in mental health. This has encouraged better recognition and treatment of anxiety, depression, and other psychiatric conditions that often co-exist with cancer. It has drawn attention to the importance of the manner in which doctors and nurses communicate with patients about diagnosis and prognosis and encouraged the teaching of skills in this area. Also, it has promoted the use of preventive interventions, such as relaxation training and group support, to help patients cope with their illness. There has also been a growth of research interest in psychoneuroimmunology, generating clinical and laboratory studies on the mind–body connection, and reviving interest in the old idea that psychosocial factors can influence disease process directly.

Greater understanding and integration between the 'orthodox' and 'holistic' approaches would seem the obvious way forward and many patients would welcome this. For example, after attending a group support programme held in an oncology unit, one woman wrote to me saying that this had been her only positive experience at the hospital and that she considered it vital for more such services to be provided to balance the unpleasantness of the medical treatments being delivered there.

However, the integrated approach might be carried too far. If the therapies become completely absorbed into the dominant mainstream, they could become just one more tool of technology being delivered in the high-pressure hospital environment, with their unique appeal and essence being diluted or lost.

## Conclusion: seeking the 'middle way'

This brief overview has highlighted some contrasts between orthodox and complementary medicine as regards the philosophy of health and healing, the evaluation of treatments, and the delivery of services. Reconciling the discipline of EBM with more intuitive, individualized approaches to healing continues to present a challenge. Enhancing cancer care with the sort of interventions described in this book calls for the best of both worlds to be combined, seeking an appropriate balance between the extremes, as in the Buddhist 'middle way'.

Chapter 2

# Evaluating complementary therapies

Janet Richardson and Karen Pilkington

## Summary

The nature and complexities of complementary therapies and their under-pinning philosophical approaches present a challenge to the research community. Debate has ensued regarding the appropriateness of applying the 'gold standard' randomized controlled trial (RCT) approach to their evaluation. Nonetheless, in an increasingly evidence-based treatment culture, healthcare professionals and people with cancer will need to have access to the best-available evidence on the effectiveness of complementary therapies. This chapter presents a summary of the current research findings, considers the methodological challenges and safety issues, and provides resources for further details.

## Introduction

Complementary and alternative medicine (CAM) can be defined as 'a group of diverse medical and health care systems, practices, and products that are not presently considered to be part of conventional medicine' (http://nccam.nih.gov/, accessed July 2006). Some therapies, for example, homeopathy, offer complete systems of assessment and treatment, whereas others complement conventional treatment with various supportive tech-niques (HL Paper 123 2000). The list of therapies included under CAM changes continually because as new approaches to healthcare emerge, those therapies that are proven to be safe and effective are adopted into the conven-tional healthcare system. Furthermore, the status and availability of comple-mentary therapies varies in different countries and is most likely to be determined by culture and context, efforts to regulate therapies, and the extent to which their use is based on evidence.

In 1995, 70% of oncology centres in England and Wales were providing some form of complementary therapy (White 1998). A postal survey that sampled over 1000 women diagnosed with breast cancer found that more than 22% had consulted a complementary practitioner 'in the previous 12 months' (Rees *et al.* 2000). The most common therapies were massage and aromatherapy, chiropractic and osteopathy, relaxation, yoga, meditation, and healing. Recent studies suggest that the extent of use of these therapies varies among countries. For example, in 2003, use of CAM was reported to be 33% for the treatment of breast cancer (vitamins most widely used) in Germany, 52% for the treatment of various cancers (vitamins most widely used) in the UK, and 39% for the treatment of various cancers (mistletoe extracts most widely used) in Switzerland (http://www.cam-cancer.org, accessed August 2006).

Reported use may vary depending on how survey questions are asked and whether they distinguish between over-the-counter purchase and treatment by a therapist. For example, a survey in the US found that 36% of respondents reported using CAM. However, when megavitamins and prayer specifically for health reasons was included in the definition of CAM, the reported use increased to 62% (http://nccam.nih.gov/news/ camsurvey_fs1.htm, accessed August 2006). Research demonstrates that people with cancer use complementary therapies to prolong survival, palliate symptoms, alleviate the side effects of conventional treatment, boost the immune system, and enhance physical and emotional well-being (Rees *et al.* 2000; Correa-Velez *et al.* 2005; Molassiotis *et al.* 2005; Humpel and Jones 2006).

People with cancer are vulnerable and, when seeking information about complementary therapies, need assurances that the therapy is of high quality and based on appropriate evidence. The Internet is a major source of information that is easily accessible but may be overwhelming in quantity. For example, a Google search in 2006 produced around 38 million hits for 'Complementary Medicine' and 139 million hits for 'Alternative Medicine'. It can be difficult for users to navigate their way towards information of the highest quality (Pilkington and Richardson 2003). Many CAM web sites encourage people to buy products that have not been independently evaluated. Others do not include relevant details or include inaccurate information. A study that analyzed 150 web sites that focused on three widely used herbs reported that 25% of the web sites contained statements that could lead to direct physical harm if acted upon and that 97% omitted vital information (Walji *et al.* 2004). A survey of CAM web sites most likely to be used by patients with cancer reported similar results (Schmidt and Ernst 2004). The authors assessed the quality of material posted on 32 web sites using predefined criteria and reported that most sites issued recommendations for a plethora of treatments that were not supported by scientific evidence. The material posted in three sites was considered to have the potential

for harming patients, while the information was generally of extremely vari-
able quality.

The objective of this chapter is to provide an overview of the benefits and risks
of complementary therapies, with further resources that will enable practitioners and researchers to access additional information if they choose to.
The focus will be on therapies that are 'complementary' (used together with)
rather than 'alternative' (used in place of) to conventional medicine.

## Research challenges

Researching complementary therapies in cancer care presents a number of
challenges, specifically those related to conducting research on patients who
may have a life-limiting illness, have associated complex emotional needs,
or require palliative care (Ingleton and Davies 2004). Issues regarding the
most appropriate research methodology for evaluating complementary therapies
add a further dimension to these challenges (Buchanan *et al.* 2005). The RCT
is the standard procedure used for investigating the effectiveness of healthcare
interventions. However, the use of RCTs in complementary therapies is
a hotly debated topic. There are a number of factors influencing this debate;
for example, the different explanatory models underpinning some complementary therapies, the 'whole systems' approach combining a range of modalities
and providing individualized treatments, and the challenges of finding suitable
placebo procedures (Richardson 2000; Verhoef *et al.* 2005; Hammerschlag and
Zwickey 2006). Positive attempts to overcome such challenges have been
proposed by a number of researchers and include the use of pragmatic clinical
trials (Richardson 2000, 2001; Macpherson 2004) and whole-systems approaches
(Verhoef *et al.* 2005). The challenges of RCTs specifically in relation to integrative
cancer care have been investigated by Block *et al.* (2004*a,b*). Consequently,
efforts to examine the evidence base for complementary therapies are hampered
by the limited number of research studies of high methodological quality that
assess interventions as they would be delivered in normal clinical practice.

## Evidence

Complementary therapies have the potential to provide some relief for the
symptoms of cancer and the side effects of treatments. These vary at different
stages of the illness, and so patients may benefit from different therapies at
different times. Finding evidence for the effectiveness of complementary
therapies presents a challenge (Pilkington and Richardson 2004; Pilkington
*et al.* 2005) and hence the list of appropriate resources at the end of this chapter.
Concrete evidence is scarce (Ernst and Cassileth 1999; Ernst 2001) due to the

limited number of clinical studies of high methodological quality. The following section focuses on the evidence obtained by recent systematic reviews on the effectiveness of complementary therapies in cancer supportive care and symptom relief. These reviews were obtained through searches of a number of sources including the Cochrane Database of Systematic Reviews, the Database of Abstracts of Reviews of Effects, the CAMEOL (CAM Evidence Online) database, and the National Library for Health Complementary and Alternative Medicine Specialist Library. A number of these reviews include a clinical commentary and details of methodological issues that affect the integrity of the intervention. Due to space limitations, such details have not been included in full in this section. Rather, this section presents a summary of the evidence and readers are encouraged to access the full reviews for further details and to check for updates as additional studies are published. Furthermore, we fully acknowledge the limitations of controlled clinical trials and the fact that they tell us little of individual patient experience. Therefore, we have included a brief paragraph on the potential contribution of qualitative research.

## Control of symptoms

### Breathlessness

A systematic review on the use of acupuncture for the treatment of breathlessness in patients with cancer (Richardson *et al.* 2005*a*) located two unpublished RCTs, one non-randomized controlled study and an uncontrolled study. These findings suggest that evidence supporting the use of acupuncture in the treatment of breathlessness in patients with cancer is currently limited and that further research is required. No adverse effects were reported in these studies but as these were small, the safety of acupuncture for the treatment of cancer patients with dyspnoea needs further investigation. One of the RCTs was published subsequently and reported breathlessness scores that were slightly higher for patients with advanced cancer receiving true versus placebo acupuncture; however, these differences were not considered clinically significant (Vickers *et al.* 2005).

### Hot flushes

The results of uncontrolled studies suggest that acupuncture may be beneficial for the alleviation of symptoms of hot flush resulting from the use of tamoxifen in women or from castration therapy in men (Smith *et al.* 2005*a*). Heterogeneity of patient characteristics, acupuncture interventions, and outcome measures make comparison between studies difficult. Flaws in the reporting of interventions and findings were present in the majority of studies. In light of the limited availability of data on controlled research, definite conclusions on efficacy cannot be drawn. No adverse effects were reported, but again studies were small and further evaluation of this aspect is required. Future research should include appropriately powered RCTs, comparisons of different acupuncture interventions, symptom severity and quality of life as outcome measures, and use of diaries, with longer periods of follow-up. Further research on males with vasomotor symptoms and the evaluation of the relevance, validity, and applicability of standardized vasomotor symptom instruments for this group are also recommended.

Black cohosh is a plant extract from the rhizome and root of *Actaea racemosa*, previously known as *Cimicifuga racemosa* (Jellin and Gregory 2003*a*). Initially it was thought to have an oestrogenic effect, thus accounting for its beneficial effects in relieving menopausal symptoms (Blumenthal *et al.* 1998; Winterhoff *et al.* 2002). However, other studies dispute this finding (Liu *et al.* 2001), with additional evidence demonstrating that extracts from black cohosh may have anti-oestrogenic activity (Zierau *et al.* 2002). A systematic review of the use of black cohosh in the treatment of patients with cancer found the results of trials to be mixed (Smith *et al.* 2005*b*). One trial reported positive effects of black cohosh on hot flushes in patients with cancer (Hernandez and Pluchino 2003), whereas another reported positive outcomes only for sweating (Jacobson *et al.* 2001). Trials suffer from methodological limitations including a high attrition rate and varied dose, together with limited reporting of details such as those on preparations used. Due to a lack of randomized clinical trials of appropriate size and quality, there is limited evidence to suggest that use of black cohosh offers significant symptom improvement compared with controls. Although several studies have focused on the safety of use of black cohosh in the treatment of patients with breast cancer, the results have not been conclusive. The National Institutes of Health Office of Dietary Supplements information sheet on black cohosh states that 'Women with breast cancer may want to avoid black cohosh until its effects on breast tissue are understood' (NIH ODS 2005). Additionally, the UK Medicines and Healthcare Products Regulatory Agency conducted a review of the safety of black cohosh particularly in relation to reports on hepatotoxicity and concluded that the data 'support a causal association between black cohosh and the risk of liver disorders' and recommended caution in its use (MHRA 2006).

A systematic review on the use of homeopathy for the treatment of cancer concluded that positive results recorded from uncontrolled studies indicate a need to conduct well-designed RCTs to examine the effectiveness of homeopathy for treatment of hot flushes in patients with breast cancer (Richardson *et al.* 2005b).

## Dry mouth problems due to chemotherapy

Several RCTs have been conducted to examine the impact of acupuncture on cancer treatment–induced dry mouth (Blom *et al.* 1992, 1996; Wong *et al.* 2003). The results were mixed, with some evidence for increased salivary production in the acupuncture group, with effects being maintained over a 3-year period and some showing improvements in both the acupuncture and placebo groups. Problems with response to 'placebo' acupuncture often cause difficulties in the interpretation of the results of acupuncture trials. Heterogeneity of patient characteristics, acupuncture interventions,and outcome measures make comparison between studies difficult. Omissions in the reporting of interventions and findings were observed in the majority of studies. Minor side effects of the therapy included small haematomas at the acupuncture point sites and fatigue following treatment. In light of the limited availability of data on controlled research and the fact that placebo acupuncture also appeared to have an effect, definite conclusions on efficacy cannot be drawn. Future research should include symptom severity and quality of life as outcome measures and provide full intervention details in study reporting.

A single RCT investigating the effect of homeopathy in chemotherapy-induced mucositis indicated that a homeopathic mouth rinse preparation may significantly reduce chemotherapy-induced mucositis in children undergoing bone marrow transplantation (Oberbaum *et al.* 2001).

## Nausea and vomiting induced by chemotherapy

A Cochrane review of acupuncture for cancer-related nausea and vomiting (Ezzo *et al.* 2006) concluded that 'electro-acupuncture has demonstrated benefit for chemotherapy-induced acute vomiting' and that 'self-administered acupressure appears to have a protective effect for acute nausea and can readily be taught to patients'. However, additional trials are required to assess acupuncture combined with 'state-of-the-art antiemetics' to assess any additional benefit(s).

Conclusions regarding the effects of homeopathy on chemotherapy-induced nausea and vomiting (CINV) cannot be drawn due to the limited reporting of study results (Richardson *et al.* 2005*b*).

Studies on hypnosis report positive results including statistically significant reductions in anticipatory nausea and vomiting and CINV. Meta-analysis has demonstrated that hypnosis could be a clinically valuable intervention for anticipatory nausea and vomiting and CINV in children with cancer (Richardson *et al.*, in press). Further research into the effectiveness, acceptance, and feasibility of hypnosis in CINV, particularly in adults, is suggested.

## Pain and painful procedures

Lee *et al.* (2005) reviewed three RCTs and four uncontrolled studies regarding the use of acupuncture for the treatment of cancer-related pain. Although one high-quality trial of ear acupuncture showed statistically significant positive results, the others had methodological limitations. Consequently, the authors concluded that the evidence currently available was insufficient to support the effectiveness of acupuncture as an adjunct analgesic method for the treatment of patients with cancer. However, they suggest that because of its widespread acceptance, appropriately powered RCTs are needed.

In a review of behavioural interventions for cancer treatment and side effects, Redd *et al.* (2001) concluded that interventions incorporating distraction had a positive impact on anxiety and distress associated with painful and diagnostic procedures and radiation therapy.

A systematic review and meta-analysis (Devine 2003) concluded that psycho-educational interventions (progressive muscular relaxation, hypnosis, and guided imagery) may be helpful as an adjunctive treatment but they should not replace conventional analgesia.

Wilde and Espie (2004) conducted a systematic review into the efficacy of hypnosis in the reduction of procedural pain and distress in children with cancer and concluded that evidence to date was not robust enough to recommend hypnosis in best-practice guidelines for procedural pain in paediatric cancer management. A subsequent systematic review (Richardson *et al.* 2006) reported positive results from use of hypnosis including statistically significant reductions in pain and anxiety in children undergoing bone marrow aspirations or lumbar punctures. Studies were small but included comparison against other therapies and no treatment. It was concluded that hypnosis has the potential to be a clinically useful intervention for procedure-related pain and distress in paediatric cancer.

## Skin reactions to radiotherapy

*Aloe vera* gel is a clear, jelly-like substance obtained from the thin-walled sticky cells of the inner portion of the leaf of the *Aloe vera* plant (Jellin and Gregory 2003*b*). It is commonly used to treat skin complaints. Studies on the effect of *Aloe vera* gel in the treatment of radiation-induced skin reactions showed mixed results or no benefit, whereas two studies found *Aloe vera* gel to be less effective than other creams (Richardson *et al.* 2005*c*). Therefore, there is currently no evidence from RCTs to suggest that topical application of *Aloe vera* gel is effective in preventing or minimizing radiation-induced skin reactions in patients with cancer. Future research should focus on assessing the effectiveness of other topical products that have the potential to reduce the adverse impact of radiotherapy on skin.

The results of two RCTs on use of homeopathy in the treatment of radiation-induced skin reactions are inconclusive (Kulkarni *et al.* 1998; Balzarini *et al.* 2000), suggesting that further research is required prior to making recommendations for clinical practice.

## Well-being

Complementary therapies are frequently used to relieve anxiety and other mood disturbances, to reduce stress, and to improve sleep. In assessing the evidence for effectiveness, such symptoms are difficult to separate, as studies are often designed to address a number of outcome measures and include a variety of measurement tools. Consequently, relevant studies are considered here under the broad heading 'well-being'.

A Cochrane review of aromatherapy and massage (Fellowes *et al.* 2004) included eight RCTs and concluded that 'massage and aromatherapy confer short-term benefits on psychological well-being, with the effect on anxiety supported by limited evidence'. The review suggested that 'effects on physical symptoms may also occur, but the evidence is mixed as to whether aromatherapy enhances the effects of massage'. The authors recommended that replication, longer follow-up, and larger trials are needed to accrue the necessary evidence.

Reflexology in patients with cancer has not yet been the subject of a systematic review. However, several clinical trials have been conducted. Three RCTs have assessed the effects of reflexology on quality of life, mood, and pain, respectively (Hodgson 2000; Ross 2002; Stephenson *et al.* 2003). A further non-randomized study assessed anxiety and pain (Stephenson *et al.* 2000). Positive results were reported; however, when reflexology was compared with non-specific foot massage, the findings were contradictory, with one study reporting a difference and the other reporting no difference. This can be attributed to the small sample size of the studies. As the interventions appeared to be well-received by patients, with the majority reporting increased relaxation, further larger-scale trials are required to fully assess the effects.

Roffe *et al.* (2005) concluded that guided imagery as an adjuvant cancer therapy may be psychosupportive and increase comfort. There is some evidence to suggest that meditation can have a positive effect on coping abilities and increase optimism and reduce the severity and duration of chemotherapy nausea (Richardson *et al.* 2005*d*). However, the small number of published clinical trials suggests that further research is required before firm conclusions can be drawn regarding clinical practice. Areas of potential research in cancer supportive care include the impact of meditation on sleep, stress, and anxiety; nausea and vomiting; emotional well-being and quality of life; and coping abilities.

Mindfulness-based stress reduction (MBSR) is a specific, highly structured psycho-educational and skill-based therapy package that combines mindfulness meditation with Hatha yoga exercises and is traditionally delivered as an 8-week programme. Studies report positive results, including improvement in mood and sleep quality, and reduction in stress. MBSR has potential as a clinically valuable, self-administered intervention for patients with cancer (Smith *et al.* 2005c). However, additional appropriately powered and rigorous RCTs investigating the efficacy, feasibility, acceptability, and safety of MBSR for patients with cancer are required.

There is some limited evidence to suggest that yoga can reduce sleep disturbance and increase emotional well-being (Richardson *et al.* 2005e). The small number of published clinical trials suggests that further research is required before firm conclusions can be drawn regarding clinical practice. Areas of potential research in cancer supportive care include the impact of yoga on sleep, stress, and anxiety; chemotherapy toxicity; emotional well-being and quality of life; and coping abilities. Furthermore, full reporting of the type of yoga intervention will make comparison and replication possible.

## Plant-based treatments for cancer

Mistletoe (*Viscum album*) extracts are among the most popular complementary therapies used in the treatment of cancer in Europe (Grothey 1998). European mistletoe is a semiparasitic plant that grows on oak, pine, elm, apple, and other trees. Three systematic reviews have focused on the use of mistletoe in the treatment of patients with cancer. Estimates of the effectiveness with regard to quality of life and survival have varied due to methodological differences but overall the findings are contradictory (Kleijnen and Knipschild 1994; Ernst *et al.* 2003; Kienle *et al.* 2003). There is little information on safety reported in these reviews, although reported side effects include inflammation at injection sites, raised temperature, chills, swelling of lymph nodes, thrombophlebitis, headache, circulatory problems, and allergic reactions including anaphylaxis (Kaegi 1998; Hutt *et al.* 2001; Loewe-Mesch 2002). On the basis of the current evidence, no definite conclusions can be drawn regarding the efficacy or safety of mistletoe for the treatment of cancer.

Essiac is a herbal tea mixture originally developed in Canada. It has been claimed that Essiac can help detoxify the body and strengthen the immune system. It is reported to contain four herbs: burdock root (*Arctium lappa*), Indian rhubarb root (*Rheum palmatum*), sheep sorrel (*Rumex acetosella*), and the inner bark of slippery elm (*Ulmus fulva* or *Ulmus rubra*). Although Essiac has received much attention in the popular press, there is currently no evidence from published clinical studies on its effectiveness in treating cancer (Pilkington and Richardson 2005).

A Cochrane review (Taixiang *et al.* 2005) of *Chinese herbs* for reduction of side effects of chemotherapy in patients with colorectal cancer found 'some evidence that decoctions of Huangqi compounds may stimulate immuno-competent cells and decrease side effects in patients treated with chemotherapy'. However, they also point to the methodological limitations of the studies and consequently conclude that there is 'no robust demonstration of benefit'. They found no evidence of harm from the use of Chinese herbs.

## What qualitative studies tell us about cancer and complementary therapies

A qualitative approach is increasingly being included in RCTs, for example, in order to investigate patient experience in greater depth or assess the integrity of the intervention. Qualitative studies are also relevant in exploring patient expectations of complementary therapies (Richardson 2004a). A review of qualitative studies that focused on the experience of patients with cancer opting for complementary therapies (Richardson *et al.* 2004b) demonstrated that the information gained from qualitative studies provides valuable information on the wider benefits of CAM treatment, the feasibility of interventions, the importance of context, and patient needs. Such richness of data provides a holistic picture of the therapies, taking into account the individual patient's experience, the notion of process, and the importance of context, including the relevance of the philosophies of the therapies.

## Risk and safety

Although often thought to be 'safe and natural', complementary therapies are not without risk. Several reviews of the safety of specific therapies have been conducted. For example, two reviews concluded that massage for patients with cancer is not entirely risk free, although serious adverse events are rare (Ernst 2003; Corbin 2005). Herbal medicines are the main focus of attention in terms of safety and have been found to be responsible for more adverse events in the elderly than acupuncture, spinal manipulation, or massage (Ernst 2002). A major concern is when patients combine the use of herbs with conventional therapy (Smith and Boon 1999). Healthcare professionals need to be aware of what complementary therapies their patients are using, or considering, in order to help them make safe and informed decisions. This requires an awareness of the potential interactions and contra-indications. Several reviews focusing on the safety of herbal medicines have been published. Boon and Wong (2004) provide a comprehensive overview of those herbs likely to be used by patients to prevent or treat cancer, or relieve adverse effects of cancer treatment. A similar review tabulates potential adverse effects of the herbs and supplements often used by patients with cancer (Werneke *et al.* 2004).

Weiger *et al.* (2002) summarized the literature on a range of CAM therapies commonly used by patients with cancer, focusing on evidence about disease progression and palliation and on the question of efficacy in addition to safety. Evidence is tabulated for individual interventions including dietary modifications, herbal products, massage, and acupuncture, showing the level of evidence, risks, and contra-indications. Details on therapies whose use should be discouraged or avoided are also provided.

Safety issues are not always evident from clinical trials or even systematic reviews as many of the studies are of small scale and adverse effects may be relatively infrequent. Therefore, ongoing safety monitoring of complementary therapies together with collation of individual reports of suspected adverse events is required. The value of this approach has been demonstrated in relation to acupuncture. There are numerous sources of information on the safety of acupuncture and it is accepted that there are potential risks associated with it, although serious adverse events are rare. Detailed information on incidence and types of adverse effects encountered in practice has been provided by a series of large-scale studies (e.g. Macpherson *et al.* 2004; Melchart *et al.* 2004; White 2004) collating events reported by patients and/or practitioners. Several considerations related to the use of acupuncture therapy in patients receiving palliative care have also been discussed (Filshie 2001). The findings of these studies provide an important source of information that would not have been readily available from RCTs. Nevertheless, there may be additional safety considerations related to the use of specific therapies in patients with cancer and specialist sources such as those listed in this chapter are therefore important.

## Conclusion

Some complementary therapies have the potential to provide supportive (such as quality of life) benefits and symptom relief in patients with cancer. Evidence for their effectiveness from RCTs is limited due to the lack of trials of high methodological quality. There is clearly a need for further research that considers the potential benefits for specific symptoms and treatment side effects, in addition to evaluating patient experience. Integration of complementary therapies into mainstream practice will need to take account of possible adverse effects and contra-indications.

## Useful resources

Complementary and Alternative Medicine Evidence Online (UK): http://www.rccm.org.uk/cameol

Complementary and Alternative Medicine Assessment in the Cancer Field (EU): http://www.cam-cancer.org/

NHS National Library for Health Complementary and Alternative Medicine Specialist Library (UK): http://www.library.nhs.uk/cam/

National Centre for Complementary and Alternative Medicine (US): http://nccam.nih.gov/

National Cancer Institute (US): http://www.cancer.gov/cancertopics/factsheet/therapy/CAM

About Herbs, Botanicals & Other Products Published by Memorial Sloan-Kettering Cancer Centre: http://www.mskcc.org/mskcc/html/11570.cfm

## References

Balzarini, A., Felisi, E., Martini, A. & De Conno, F. 2000, Efficacy of homeopathic treatment of skin reactions during radiotherapy breast cancer: a randomized, double-blind clinical trial, *British Homeopathic Journal*, vol. **89**, no. 1, pp. 8–12.

Block, K. I., Burns, B. L., Cohen, A. J., Dobs, A. S., Hess, S. M. & Vickers, A. 2004*a*, Point-counterpoint: using randomized trials for the evaluation of integrative cancer therapies, *Integrative Cancer Therapies*, vol. **1**, no. 1, pp. 66–81.

Block, K. I., Cohen, A. J., Dobs, A. S. & Ornish, D. 2004*b*, The challenges of randomized trials in integrative cancer care, *Integrative Cancer Therapies*, vol. **3**, no. 2, pp. 112–27.

Blom, M., Dawidson, I. & Angmar-Mansson, B. 1992, The effect of acupuncture on salivary flow rates in patients with xerostomia, *Oral Surgery, Oral Medicine, and Oral Pathology*, vol. **73**, pp. 293–8.

Blom, M., Dawidson, I., Fernberg, J.-O., Johnson, G. & Angmar-Mansson, B. 1996, Acupuncture treatment of patients with radiation-induced xerostomia, *Oral Oncology, European Journal of Cancer*, vol. **32B**, no. 3, pp. 182–90.

Blumenthal, M., Busse, W. R. Goldberg, A. *et al.* 1998, *The complete German commission E monographs: therapeutic guide to herbal medicines*. Austin, TX: American Botanical Council.

Boon, H. & Wong, J. 2004, Botanical medicine and cancer: a review of the safety and efficacy, *Expert Opinion on Pharmacotherapy*, vol. **5**, pp. 2485–501.

Buchanan, D. R., White, J. D., O'Mara, A. M., Kelaghan, J. W., Smith, W. B. & Minasian, L. M. 2005, Research design issues in cancer symptom management trials using complementary and alternative medicine: lessons from the National Cancer Institute Community Oncology Programme experience, *Journal of Clinical Oncology*, vol. **23**, no. 27, pp. 6682–9.

Correa-Velez, I., Clavarino, A. & Eastwood, H. 2005, Surviving, relieving, repairing, and boosting up: reasons for using complementary/alternative medicine among patients with advanced cancer: a thematic analysis, *Journal of Palliative Medicine*, vol. **8**, no. 5, pp. 953–61.

Corbin, L. 2005, Safety and efficacy of massage therapy for patients with cancer. *Cancer Control*, vol. **12**, no. 3, pp. 158–64.

Devine, E. C. 2003, Meta-analysis of the effect of psychoeducational interventions on pain in adults with cancer, *Oncology Nursing Forum*, vol. **30**, no. 1, pp. 75–89.

Ernst, E. 2001, Complementary therapies in palliative cancer care, *Cancer*, vol. **91**, no. 11, pp. 2181–5.

Ernst, E. 2002, Adverse effects of unconventional therapies in the elderly: a systematic review of recent literature, *Journal of American Aging Association*, vol. **25**, pp. 11–20.

Ernst, E. 2003, The safety of massage therapy, *Rheumatology*, vol. **42**, no. 9, pp. 1101–06.

Ernst, E. & Cassileth, B. R. 1999, How useful are unconventional cancer treatments?, *European Journal of Cancer*, vol. **35**, no. 11, pp. 1608–13.

Ernst, E., Schmidt, K., & Steuer-Vogt, M. K. 2003, Mistletoe for cancer? A systematic review of randomised clinical trials, *International Journal of Cancer*, vol. **107**, no. 2, 262–7.

Ezzo, J. M. *et al.* 2006, Acupuncture-point stimulation for chemotherapy-induced nausea or vomiting, *Cochrane Database of Systematic Reviews* 2006, Issue 2. Art. No.: CD002285. DOI: 10.1002/14651858.CD002285.pub2.

Fellowes, D., Barnes, K. & Wilkinson, S. 2004, Aromatherapy and massage for symptom relief in patients with cancer, *Cochrane Database of Systematic Reviews* 2004, Issue 3. Art. No.: CD002287. DOI: 10.1002/14651858.CD002287.pub2.

Filshie, J. 2001, Safety issues of acupuncture in palliative care, *Acupuncture in Medicine: Special Safety Issue* 19(2), pp. 117–122. Available at: http://www.medical-acupuncture.co.uk/journal/2001(2)/contents.shtml

Grothey, A., Duppe, J., Hasenburg, A. & Voigtmann, R. 1998, Use of alternative medicine in oncology patients, *Deutsche medizinische Wochenschrift*, vol. **123**, nos. 31–32, pp. 923–9.

Hammerschlag, R. & Zwickey, H. 2006, Evidence-based complementary and alternative medicine: back to basics, *Journal of Alternative and Complementary Medicine*, vol. **12**, no. 4, pp. 349–50.

Hernandez, M. G. & Pluchino, S. 2003, *Cimicifuga racemosa* for the treatment of hot flushes in women surviving breast cancer, *Maturitas: The European Menopause Journal*, vol. **44**, Suppl. no. 1, pp. S59–S65.

HL Paper 123 2000, *House of Lords Select Committee on Science and Technology: Complementary and Alternative Medicine*. London: The Stationary Office.

Hodgson, H. 2000, Does reflexology impact on cancer patients' quality of life?, *Nursing Standard*, vol. **14**, no. 31, pp. 33–8.

Humpel, N. & Jones, S. C. 2006, Gaining insight into the what, why and where of complementary and alternative medicine use by cancer patients and survivors, *European Journal of Cancer Care*, vol. **15**, no. 4, pp. 326–8.

Hutt, N., Kopferschmitt-Kubler, M., Cabalion, J., Purohit, A., Alt, M. & Pauli, G. 2001, Anaphylactic reactions after therapeutic injection of mistletoe (*Viscum album* L), *Allergologia et Immunopathologia*, vol. **29**, no. 5, pp. 201–03.

Ingleton, C. & Davies, S. 2004, Research and scholarship in palliative care nursing. In *Palliative Care Nursing*, (eds) S. Payne, J. Seymour, C. Ingleton, Open University Press, Berkshire, England. pp. 688–9.

Jacobson, J. *et al.* 2001, Randomized trial of black cohosh for the treatment of hot flashes among women with a history of breast cancer, *Journal of Clinical Oncology*, vol. **19**, no. 10, pp. 2739–45.

Jellin, J. M. & Gregory, P. J. 2003a, Black cohosh. In *Natural Medicines Comprehensive Database*, 5th edn. Stockton CA: Therapeutic Research Faculty. pp. 163–5.

Jellin, J. M. & Gregory, P. J. 2003b, Aloe gel. In *Natural Medicines Comprehensive Database*, 5th edn. Stockton CA: Therapeutic Research Faculty. pp. 39–41.

Kaegi, E. 1998, Unconventional therapies for cancer: 3. Iscador. Task Force on Alternative Therapies of the Canadian Breast Cancer Research Initiative, *Canadian Medical Association Journal*, vol. **158**, no. 9, pp. 1157–9.

Kienle, G. S., Berrino, F., Bussing, A., Portalupi, E., Rosenzweig, S. & Kiene, H. 2003, Mistletoe in cancer - a systematic review on controlled clinical trials, *European Journal of Medical Research*, vol. **8**, no. 3, pp. 109–19.

Kleijnen, J. & Knipschild, P. 1994, Mistletoe treatment for cancer: review of controlled trials in humans, *Phytomedicine*, vol. **1**, 255–60.

Kulkarni, A., Nagarkar, B. M. & Burde, G. S. 1988, Radiation protection by use of homoeopathic medicines, *Hahnemannian Homoeopathic Sandesh*, vol. **12**, no. 1, pp. 20–3.

Lee, H., Schmidt, K. & Ernst, E. 2005, Acupuncture for the relief of cancer-related pain: a systematic review, *European Journal of Pain*, vol. **9**, no. 4, pp. 437–44.

Liu, J., Burdette, J. E. & Xu, H. *et al.* 2001, Evaluation of estrogenic activity of plant extracts for the potential treatment of menopausal symptoms, *Journal of Agricultural and Food Chemistry*, vol. **49**, pp. 2472–9.

Loewe-Mesch, A. 2002, Die Misteltherapie in der biologischen Tumorbegleitbehandlung - im Spannungsfeld zwischen Erfahrung und Forschungsergebnissen, *Erfahrungsheilkunde*, vol. **51**, no. 4, 256–8.

MacPherson, H. 2004, Pragmatic clinical trials, *Complementary Therapies in Medicine*, vol. **12**, pp. 136–40.

Macpherson, H., Scullion, A., Thomas, K. J. & Walters, S. 2004, Patient reports of adverse events associated with acupuncture treatment: a prospective national survey, *Quality & Safety in Health Care*, vol. **13**, no. 5, pp. 349–55.

Melchart, D., Weidenhammer, W., Streng, A., Reitmayr, S., Hoppe, A., Ernst, E. & Linde, K. 2004, Prospective investigation of adverse effects of acupuncture in 97733 patients, *Archives of Internal Medicine*, vol. **164**, no. 1, pp. 104–5.

MHRA (Medicines and Healthcare products Regulatory Agency). *Black cohosh (Cimicifuga racemosa) – risk of liver problems.* Herbal Safety News: current safety issues, July 2006. Available at: http://www.mhra.gov.uk

Molassiotis, A., Fernadez-Ortega, P., Pud, D. *et al.* 2005, Use of complementary and alternative medicine in cancer patients: a European survey, *Annals of Oncology*, vol. **16**, pp. 655–63.

NIH ODS (National Institutes of Health, Office of Dietary Supplements). *Questions and Answers About Black Cohosh and the Symptoms of Menopause.* Available at: http://ods.od.nih.gov/factsheets/BlackCohosh.asp#h10 (accessed January 19, 2005).

Oberbaum, M., Yaniv, I., Ben-Gal, Y., Stein, J., Ben-Zvi, N., Freedman, L. S. & Branski, D. 2001, A randomized controlled clinical trial of the homeopathic medication TRAUMEEL S in the treatment of chemotherapy-induced stomatitis in children undergoing stem cell transplantation, *Cancer*, vol. **92**, no. 3, pp. 684–90.

Pilkington, K. & Richardson, J. 2003, Evidence-based complementary and alternative medicine on the Internet, *He@lth Information on the Internet*, vol. **34**, pp. 7–9.

Pilkington, K. & Richardson, J. 2004, Exploring the evidence: the challenges of searching for research on acupuncture, *Journal of Complementary and Alternative Medicine*, vol. **10**, no. 3, pp. 587–90.

Pilkington, K. & Richardson, J. 2005, Essiac in cancer: a review of the evidence, *Complementary and Alternative Medicine Evidence Online (CAMEOL) Database.* Available at: http://rccm.org.uk/cameol/Default.aspx

Pilkington, K., Boshnakova, A., Clarke, M. & Richardson, J. 2005, No language restrictions in database searches: what does this really mean? *Journal of Complementary and Alternative Medicine*, vol. **11**, no. 1, pp. 205–07.

Redd, W. H., Montgomery, G. H. & DuHamel, K. N. 2001, Behavioral intervention for cancer treatment side effects, *Journal of the National Cancer Institute*, vol. **93**, no. 11, pp. 810–23.

Rees, R. W., Feigel, I., Vickers, A., Zollman, C., McGurk, R. & Smith, C. 2000, Prevalence of complementary therapy use by women with breast cancer: a population-based survey, *European Journal of Cancer*, vol. **36**, pp. 1359–64.

Richardson, J. 2000, The use of randomized control trials in complementary therapy: Exploring the methodological issues, *Journal of Advanced Nursing*, vol. **32**, no. 2, pp. 398–406.

Richardson, J. 2001, Developing and evaluating complementary therapy services. Part 2. Examining the effect of treatment on health status, *Journal of Alternative and Complementary Medicine*, vol. **7**, no. 4, pp. 315–28.

Richardson, J. 2004a, What patients expect from complementary therapy: a qualitative study, *American Journal of Public Health*, vol. **94**, pp. 1049–53.

Richardson, J., Smith, J. & Pilkington, K. 2004b, Qualitative research in complementary therapies: is it of any value?, *FACT (Focus on Alternative and Complementary Therapies)*, vol. **9**, no. 1, p. 43.

Richardson, J., Smith, J. & Pilkington, K. 2005a, Acupuncture for cancer-related breathlessness: a systematic review, *Complementary and Alternative Medicine Evidence Online (CAMEOL) Database.* Available at: http://rccm.org.uk/cameol/Default.aspx

Richardson, J., Smith, J., Kassab, S. & Pilkington, K. 2005b, Homeopathy for cancer supportive care. *Complementary and Alternative Medicine Evidence Online (CAMEOL) Database.* Available at: http://rccm.org.uk/cameol/Default.aspx

Richardson, J., Smith, J., McIntyre, M., Thomas, R. & Pilkington, K. 2005c, Aloe vera for preventing radiation-induced skin reactions: a systematic literature review, *Clinical Oncology*, vol. **17**, no. 6, pp. 478–84.

Richardson, J., Smith, J., Hoffman, C. & Pilkington, K. 2005d, Meditation as a supportive therapy in cancer: a systematic review, *Complementary and Alternative Medicine Evidence Online (CAMEOL) Database.* Available at: http://rccm.org.uk/cameol/Default.aspx

Richardson, J., Smith, J., Hoffman, C. & Pilkington, K. 2005e, Yoga as a supportive therapy in cancer. *Complementary and Alternative Medicine Evidence Online (CAMEOL) Database.* Available at: http://rccm.org.uk/cameol/Default.aspx

Richardson, J., Smith, J., McCall, G. & Pilkington, K. 2006, Hypnosis for procedure-related pain and distress in paediatric cancer patients: a systematic literature review, *Journal of Pain and Symptom Management*, vol. **31**, no. 1, pp. 70–84.

Richardson, J., Smith, J., McCall, G., Richardson, A., Pilkington, K. & Kirsch, I. Hypnosis for nausea and vomiting in cancer chemotherapy: a systematic review of the research evidence. *European Journal of Cancer Care*, in press.

Roffe, L., Schmidt, K. & Ernst, E. 2005, A systematic review of guided imagery as an adjuvant cancer therapy, *Psychooncology*, vol. **14**, no. 8, pp. 607–17.

Ross, C. 2002, A pilot study to evaluate the effect of reflexology on mood and symptom rating of advanced cancer patients, *Palliative Medicine*, vol. **16**, no. 6, pp. 544–5.

Schmidt, K. & Ernst, E. 2004, Assessing websites on complementary and alternative medicine for cancer, *Annals of Oncology*, vol. **15**, pp. 733–42.

Smith, J., Richardson, J., Filshie, J., Thomas, R., Moir, F. & Pilkington, K. 2005*a*, Acupuncture for hot flushes as a result of cancer treatment: a systematic review. *Complementary and Alternative Medicine Evidence Online (CAMEOL) Database*. Available at: http://rccm.org.uk/cameol/Default.aspx

Smith, J., Richardson, J., McIntyre, M., Thomas, R. & Pilkington, K. 2005*b*, Black cohosh for menopausal symptoms in women with breast cancer: a systematic review. *Complementary and Alternative Medicine Evidence Online (CAMEOL) Database*. Available at: http://rccm.org.uk/cameol/Default.aspx

Smith, J., Richardson, J., Hoffman, C. & Pilkington, K. 2005*c*, Mindfulness Based Stress Reduction (MBSR) as supportive therapy in cancer care: a systematic review, *Journal of Advanced Nursing*, vol. **52**, no. 3, pp. 315–27.

Smith, M. & Boon, H. 1999, Counseling cancer patients about herbal medicine, *Patient Education and Counseling*, vol. **38**, pp. 109–20.

Stephenson, N., Dalton, J. A. & Carlson, J. 2003, The effect of foot reflexology on pain in patients with metastatic cancer, *Applied Nursing Research*, vol. **16**, no. 4, pp. 284–6.

Stephenson, N. I., Weinrich, S. P. & Tavakoli, A. S. 2000, The effects of foot reflexology on anxiety and pain in patients with breast and lung cancer, *Oncology Nursing Forum*, vol. **27**, no. 1, pp. 67–72.

Taixiang, W., Munro, A. J. & Guanjian, L. 2005, Chinese medical herbs for chemotherapy side effects in colorectal cancer patients. *Cochrane Database of Systematic Reviews*. 2005 Issue 1. Art. No.: CD004540. DOI: 10.1002/1465185.CD004540.pub2.

Verhoef, M. J., Lewith, G., Ritenbaugh, C., Boon, H., Fleishman, S. & Leis, A. 2005, Complementary and alternative medicine whole systems research: beyond identification of inadequacies of the RCT, *Complementary Therapies in Medicine*, vol. **13**, pp. 206–12.

Vickers, A. J., Feinstein, M. B., Deng, G. E. & Cassileth, B. R. 2005, Acupuncture for dyspnea in advanced cancer: a randomized, placebo-controlled pilot trial, *BMC Palliative Care*, vol. **18**, pp. 4:5.

Walji, M., Sagaram, S., Sagaram, D., Meric-Bernstam, F., Johnson, C., Mirza, N. Q. & Bernstam, E. V. 2004, Efficacy of quality criteria to identify potentially harmful information: a cross-sectional survey of complementary and alternative medicine web sites, *Journal of Medical Internet Research*, vol. **6**, no. 2, p. e21.

Weiger, W. A., Smith, P., Boon, H., Richardson, M. A., Kaptchuck, T. J. & Eisenberg, D. M. 2002, Advising patients who seek complementary and alternative medical therapies for cancer, *Annals of Internal Medicine*, vol. **137**, no. 11, pp. 889–903.

Werneke, U., Ladenheim, D. & McCarthy, T. 2004, Complementary alternative medicine for cancer: a review of effectiveness and safety, *Cancer Therapy*, vol. **2**, pp. 475–500.

White, P. 1998, Complementary medicine treatment of cancer: a survey of provision, *Complementary Therapies in Medicine*, vol. **6**, pp. 10–13.

White, A. 2004, A cumulative review of the range and incidence of significant adverse events associated with acupuncture, *Acupuncture in Medicine*, vol. **22**, no. 3, pp. 122–33.

Wild, M. R. & Espie, C. A. 2004, The efficacy of hypnosis in the reduction of procedural pain and distress in pediatric oncology: a systematic review, *Journal of Developmental and Behavioral Pediatrics*, vol. **25**, pp. 207–13.

Winterhoff, H., Butterweck, V., Jarry, H. & Wuttke, W. 2002, Pharmacologic and clinical studies using cimicifuga racemosa in climacteric complaints, *Weiner Medizinische Wochenschrift*, vol. **152**, pp. 360–63. (in German)

Wong, R. K. W., Jones, G. W., Sagar. S. M., Babjak, A. -F. & Whelan, T. 2003, A phase I-II study in the use of acupuncture-like transcutaneous nerve stimulation in the treatment of radiation-induced xerostomia in head and neck cancer patients treated with radical radiotherapy, *International Radiation Oncology*, vol. **57**, no. 2, pp. 472–80.

Zierau, O., Bodinet, C., Kolba, S. *et al.* 2002, Antiestrogenic activities of Cimicifuga racemosa extracts, *Journal of Steroid Biochemistry and Molecular Biology*, vol. **80**, pp. 125–30.

Chapter 3

# The oncology setting

Teresa E Young

## Summary

As more cancer patients use complementary therapies to control symptoms and improve their quality of life, provision, both independently funded and within a state funded health system is on the increase. Setting up services to provide high-quality therapies presents a number of challenges. Liaison and communication are needed to provide an integrated service where both patients and health professionals feel reassured. Consideration should be given not only to which therapies are offered but also to how the service is promoted and delivered. Educating practitioners about cancer and its treatment is essential. Linking research to service delivery increases credibility and helps develop an evidence base.

## Introduction

For many patients in the Western world, access to complementary therapies was previously confined to those who were able to afford private treatments. However, an increasing number of countries are slowly beginning to introduce such therapies into their state-funded health system, making them accessible to a wider population at low or no cost. This trend is particularly apparent in the field of oncology, especially palliative care.

There is recognition that caring for a patient with cancer does not just involve the administration of anti-cancer treatments such as radiotherapy and chemotherapy. It is also necessary to provide a range of other treatments and services to help with physical symptoms and psychosocial issues. This is often referred to as 'supportive care' and in the UK, the National Institute for Clinical Excellence recently published guidelines for Supportive Care for Adults with Cancer (NICE 2004). Although the guidelines do not actually recommend complementary therapies (due to lack of evidence), they do acknowledge that many patients express an interest in these therapies to help them deal with physical symptoms and psychological distress. The guidelines stress the need for high-quality information to help patients make decisions. They also recommend that 'Provider organisations should ensure that any practitioner delivering complementary therapies in NHS settings conforms to policies designed to ensure best practice ...' (p. 151).

This chapter focuses on one such provider organization—the Lynda Jackson Macmillan Centre (LJMC)—and will discuss some of the challenges encountered during the past 13 years in setting up and maintaining a 'drop-in' support and information centre. LJMC is located in the building adjacent to a large regional cancer treatment centre—Mount Vernon Cancer Centre (MVCC)—which serves a population of 2 million living north-west of central London. MVCC has more than 25 consultant oncologists who visit 15 district general hospitals, where most of the cancer surgery is performed. Patients then travel to MVCC for chemotherapy and/or radiotherapy. The complementary therapies initially provided by LJMC were aromatherapy, reflexology, Alexander technique, shiatsu, and relaxation classes. More recently, Reiki, acupuncture, ear acupuncture, and Indian head massage have been introduced. These are provided by both paid and volunteer therapists with previous experience of working with patients with cancer. In addition, LJMC provides counselling, 'supportive listening' from trained volunteers and health professionals, and a wealth of information about cancer and its treatments (both orthodox and complementary) in the form of leaflets, books, videos, etc. From the outset, the choice of therapies and services offered has been heavily influenced by 'user involvement' (Howells *et al.* 1998) and there is an ongoing research and evaluation programme.

## Integration

LJMC is now considered an integral part of the Cancer Treatment Centre and is funded partially by the National Health Service (NHS) and partially by voluntary donations. LJMC has representation on the Board of the Cancer Treatment Centre and at clinical governance meetings. The key to the successful integration has been a liaison to ensure that LJMC has the respect and support of the staff in the cancer treatment centre, including doctors, nurses, and therapy radiographers. Measures taken to achieve this are discussed below.

### Complementary, not alternative

LJMC acts both as a provider of complementary therapies and as an information resource for patients, carers, and health professionals about complementary and alternative therapies. Although LJMC does hold information about alternative treatments, all the services provided at LJMC are promoted as complementary and not alternative to orthodox treatment. However the centre does hold information about alternative treatments and this will be given to patients upon request. The emphasis is on providing patients with information to help them make their own informed choice and not on recommending or dismissing a particular therapy. The first person to greet callers to LJMC is often a volunteer trained in 'supportive listening'. However, if patients are seeking medical advice or information on safety and efficacy of complementary therapies, a trained health professional is always on call. They can discuss with patients any leaflets held by LJMC that contain complex, sensitive, or contentious medical advice and which are likely to stimulate further questions. This system prevents accusations of paternalism and 'gate-keeping' while giving the medical staff the confidence to refer their patients to LJMC for advice.

As part of a study recently undertaken jointly by LJMC and the Cancer Treatment Centre at Southampton (Corner *et al.* 2006), patients were asked reasons for using or not using complementary therapies. Endorsement by their consultant was often seen as the key:

'... I also have not been advised by my "cancer doctor" if any or some CAM would be beneficial. I would seek his advice first of all and be guided'

'I was encouraged to use CAM by the Macmillan nurse attending me and also my doctor'

However, they also mentioned that they were confused when one health professional was recommending a particular therapy, whereas others were concerned as to its safety and efficacy:

'... I asked advice (about hot flushes) when attending radiotherapy. First one said evening primrose oil—another later suggested if it didn't work try extract of sage ... . I personally think the primrose oil is beginning to help but I had a call from one of the breast nurses recently and according to her it's a waste of time! Confusing or what?'

'Choice was, however, restricted as I found the medical profession reluctant for me to undertake anything—especially to take any supplements that I had read about to help whilst undergoing treatment'

There is a dilemma for health professionals too. Due to the lack of published research, systematic reviews, such as those carried out under the auspices of the Cochrane Review Collaboration, are often inconclusive and unable to reach a recommendation, except that more research is needed; yet, patients see their consultant as a source of advice. In these circumstances, the LJMC is able to provide the time and expertise to discuss with patients the sometimes limited evidence that is available.

## Experiential sessions

LJMC runs experiential workshops for patients, where they are able to try aromatherapy massage, reflexology, and Indian head massage. In addition, staff are encouraged to try out therapies themselves so that they can describe the experience to their patients.

## Communication

On completion of a course of complementary therapy, letters are sent to the patient's consultant oncologist and general practitioner. This practice reinforces the message that complementary therapy is an integral part of cancer care and it maintains a high profile for the service.

## Training

All therapists working at LJMC, whether paid or volunteer, have training and accreditation in their chosen therapy. In addition, they have to attend a 2-day workshop entitled 'Cancer and its Treatments' and 'Using Complementary Therapies with Cancer Patients'. The workshop is run on a regular basis and is also open to therapists already working in the local area in a cancer environment and to those who are considering starting. The first day covers basic medical information about cancer. Information is provided on orthodox treatments such as surgery, chemotherapy, radiotherapy, hormone therapy, and immunotherapy. Participants are shown examples of different scans such as magnetic resonance imaging, computed tomography, and ultrasound and are given a brief explanation about clinical trials and other research projects. On the second day, the therapists are led along the patients' journey, discussing the various stages of disease from diagnosis through treatment, remission, relapse, and the palliative phase. Information is given about common symptoms and side effects experienced by patients with cancer. The session also covers contra-indications to complementary therapy and safety issues specific to patients with cancer, and an experienced therapist speaks about what it is like to work with patients with cancer on the wards and in the clinics. The final afternoon involves practical sessions. To help the therapists gain real-time experience, patients from the cancer centre and local support groups are invited to sample the different therapies. During the course, attendees are 'vetted' to ensure that they are not expressing unrealistic expectations about complementary therapies 'curing' cancer. Therapists should also be empathic with patients with cancer and not have had a recent personal experience of cancer or a bereavement among their family or friends, which may leave them emotionally vulnerable.

## Network of therapists

In order that patients may continue to receive complementary therapies near their homes once their course of treatment at LJMC is completed, a network of therapists has been established. To be eligible to join the network, therapists must have attended the workshop described earlier. As they are working in their own private practice, they usually charge fees, although sometimes at a reduced rate. Some are able to offer home visits. Evening and weekend workshops are organized for network members, and there are updates on new cancer treatments and techniques.

## Involvement in research

An ongoing research programme to evaluate the complementary therapies and services, leading to scientific publications, enhances the reputation of LJMC and maintains credibility with health professionals.

# Service delivery

## Appointments

Patients may be referred by a health professional, or may self-refer, for complementary therapy at any point along their cancer journey. They may be newly diagnosed, on treatment, in remission, long-term survivors, had recent relapse, receiving palliative treatment, or in the terminal phase of illness. Their requirements and mobility will differ according to the stage of disease. Therefore, it is important to ensure that they are informed as soon as possible of the services available and have a flexible appointment system.

Patients often talk about not feeling 'in control' when it comes to their cancer treatment. They view choosing to have a complementary therapy, whether it is a body works massage type therapy, a relaxation class, or an 'over-the-counter' product as a means of regaining some control. For some patients, it is an active choice. They may have been using a particular complementary therapy prior to the diagnosis of cancer and may wish to continue with the same. For other patients, complementary therapy may be a new experience that was offered initially as a free service.

*'I used CAM as it was offered and I had never had it before, having never tried it before and it was free I had nothing to lose'*

Such patients may initially regard the therapy as a 'nice treat' and enjoy the personalized attention but they do not necessarily see it as an important and integral part of their cancer treatment. They may not value an appointment for a complementary therapy in the same way they would value one for a scan or a clinic visit. For those who do not live near the hospital, travelling is often quite stressful. Some patients use hospital transport, others rely upon friends or relatives. But once their active anti-cancer treatment is completed, additional journeys to the hospital for complementary therapies may not be a priority, although research suggests that the period between the last treatment and the first follow-up appointment (usually at 6 weeks following radiotherapy) is the one during which patients feel particularly vulnerable.

When LJMC first opened in 1993, all patients requesting aromatherapy were offered a course of six 1-hour appointments at weekly intervals, booked at the outset, taking place in dedicated rooms in LJMC. However, an audit of the first 63 patients revealed that only two-thirds had completed all six sessions (Kite *et al.* 1998). Inpatients, those with advanced disease, and those with poor performance status rarely completed more than one or two sessions. Moreover, many had failed to cancel their appointments and DNAs (Did Not Attend) are frustrating when a service is funded at least in part by voluntary donations and there is a waiting list. Therefore, a new, more flexible system was introduced and the service was split into three:

1  A 'rapid response' team, mostly volunteers, was allocated to the inpatients. Therapists visit the ward each day and offer a single session of aromatherapy or reflexology to any patient there. These patients are often less ambulatory than those who 'drop-in' to LJMC and may be in the later phases of their cancer journey. They may not be able to commit to regular outpatient appointments.

2  Meanwhile, other therapists work in the drop-in centre. Patients who are able to visit the centre and appear to be in reasonably good health are put on the waiting list and then offered up to four appointments, often at weekly intervals. (Appointments can also be arranged to fit around chemotherapy schedules at 3 weekly intervals. Some patients report that this helps control their nausea, fatigue, and lack of energy.) These sessions take place in dedicated rooms in LJMC and may include aromatherapy, reflexology, Indian head massage, or Reiki. Patients are asked to give 24 hours notice if they are unable to attend and a small deposit is taken that is returnable on completion of the full course.

3  Finally, if therapists know they have no appointments booked and there are no ward patients requesting therapy, they will visit the outpatient waiting areas in chemotherapy and radiotherapy and offer patients a hand massage or an Indian head massage in a private room nearby.

On a subsequent re-audit, the number of sessions lost to DNAs had been significantly reduced. Ward staff reported that patients appreciated the therapies being delivered at the bedside and often slept much better the following night. The chemotherapy nurses also reported that cannulation was easier for some patients and that radiotherapy patients requiring facial moulds were more relaxed.

## Choice of therapies

The choice of therapies offered in an oncology setting will be determined by a number of factors including patients' symptoms, therapists' experience, space

**Table 3.1** Reasons for referral as judged by health professional and patient-therapist

|  | Reason for referral (health professional) (%) | Rank | Symptom assessment (patient and therapist) (%) | Rank |
|---|---|---|---|---|
| Tension | 47 | 1 | 48 | 1 |
| Stress | 40 | 2 | 31 | 6 |
| Anxiety/fear | 40 | 2 | 38 | 4 |
| Tiredness | 21 | 4 | 36 | 5 |
| Insomnia | 17 | 5 | 45 | 2 |
| Pain | 16 | 6 | 40 | 3 |
| Depression | 16 | 7 | 8 | 8 |
| Physical exhaustion | 5 | 8 | 19 | 7 |

considerations, any ongoing research or evaluation, and patients' own preferences. The most common reasons for referral to LJMC are anxiety, mild depression, muscle tension, tiredness, fatigue, pain, insomnia, headaches, constipation, and nausea. The reasons for referral as judged by health professionals and the symptoms identified at assessment by the patient and therapist in a sample of 89 consecutive patients at the centre (Kite *et al.* 1998) are given in Table 3.1.

Ideally, patients who are offered a course of therapy will be briefly assessed when they first 'drop-in' to LJMC. If this is not possible, patients are telephoned at home. A decision will then be made as to the most appropriate treatment to offer. A chart (Table 3.2) is used to guide the choice. A full assessment is then undertaken by the therapist at the first treatment appointment.

## Relaxation classes

In addition to the therapies, LJMC runs 'drop-in' relaxation classes at fixed times each week. No appointment is necessary and carers are welcome, space permitting. Patients are taught breathing and relaxation techniques along with visualization and are encouraged to practise their new skills at home. Tapes and CDs are made available.

As part of an evaluation of the relaxation classes and the aromatherapy massage service, a series of focus groups was convened. Patients enjoyed the group environment of a relaxation class and spoke about the active participation required when compared with the more passive role they were able to adopt while having aromatherapy massage. Motivation was another issue raised.

**Table 3.2** Guideline chart for choosing appropriate complementary therapies

| Indications for referral | Indian head massage | Massage | Aromatherapy | Reflexology | Reiki | Ear acupuncture (tamoxifen related symptoms) | Relaxation/ visualization classes |
|---|---|---|---|---|---|---|---|
| Patient preference | ✓ | ✓ | ✓ | ✓ | ✓ | ✓ | ✓ |
| Unwillingness to undress | ✓ | | | ✓ | ✓ | | ✓ |
| Anxiety | ✓ | ✓ | ✓ | ✓ | ✓ | ✓ | ✓✓✓ |
| Depression (mild) | ✓ | ✓ | ✓ | ✓ | ✓ | | ✓ |
| Muscle tension | ✓✓ | ✓✓✓ | ✓✓✓ | | | | ✓✓ |
| Tiredness | ✓ | ✓ | ✓ | ✓✓ | ✓ | ✓ | ✓ |
| Extreme exhaustion/weakness | ✓ | ✓ | ✓ | ✓ | ✓✓ | | |
| Extreme pain e.g., bone pain | | | | | ✓✓ | | |
| Insomnia | ✓ | ✓ | ✓ | ✓ | ✓ | ✓ | ✓ |
| Headaches | ✓✓ | ✓ | ✓✓ | ✓✓✓ | ✓ | | ✓ |
| Constipation | ✓ | ✓ | ✓✓ | ✓✓✓ | | | |
| Nausea | ✓ | ✓ | ✓ | ✓ | ✓ | | ✓ |
| Hot flushes | | | | ✓ | | ✓✓✓ | |

An individual appointment booked with a personal therapist for aromatherapy massage was seen by some as an incentive to get out of their house. Initially, there was less incentive to attend a group relaxation class where you would not be missed if you did not attend. Therefore, the motivation for attending a relaxation class was the desire to meet other people and learn a new skill to help with self-management—for some this motivation only comes with time.

## Research and development

Evidence for the effectiveness of many complementary therapies is lacking and a key recommendation of the House of Lords Report (House of Lords 2000) and various grant-awarding bodies is that more research should be undertaken. Within LJMC, there is a policy that the choice of new therapies should be patient-led and that no new therapies shall be introduced unless they are evaluated or included in a research project.

### Acupuncture and ear acupuncture

As patients attend the drop-in centre, the reason for their visit is logged. This data is analyzed annually to ensure that the services provided meet the demands of the patients. An increasingly common request was for help in controlling hot flushes experienced as a side effect of taking adjuvant tamoxifen as a treatment for early breast cancer. Conventional treatments such as hormone replacement therapy are not recommended in this patient population and concerns have been raised about the safety of herbal remedies such as black cohosh. There is a range of pharmacological options available on prescription but many women are reluctant to take them. A literature search suggested that acupuncture might be effective in controlling menopausal hot flushes but the studies were all small and poorly reported. A small survey was therefore conducted on consecutive patients in the centre to establish the severity of the problem and to ensure that there would be sufficient patients willing to receive traditional acupuncture if it were offered. A research acupuncturist then prepared a protocol to evaluate traditional acupuncture for this condition and the project was promoted to the consultant oncologists and breast care nurses in the cancer centre. Patients could only receive the therapy if they consented to join the study. They were expected to complete hot flush diaries and other questionnaires before, during, and after treatment. After the study closed, participants were invited to take part in focus groups to gain qualitative data on their experiences. Once 50 patients had been recruited, their data were analyzed and the treatment and the results appeared promising (de Valois *et al.* 2002, 2003). However, concerns were expressed at the complexity of this approach, which is dynamic and changes as the patient's health changes, thus affecting the feasibility of offering it as a service without some modification.

To attempt to meet the high demand, the research acupuncturist considered using ear acupuncture delivered according to the National Acupuncture Detoxification Association (NADA) protocol (Brumbaugh 1994). Although this protocol was primarily developed to treat detoxification symptoms in substance abusers, both mapping the ear acupuncture points to acupuncture points and anecdotal evidence suggested it might be a suitable treatment for hot flushes. It has the potential advantage that it is usually delivered in a group setting. A small pilot study was conducted with six women who had previously received the traditional acupuncture treatment and they were invited to share their experiences and contribute to the design of a second protocol. In particular, their views on having needles placed in their ears and being seen in a group environment were sought. An additional 50 patients were then treated with ear acupuncture in groups of approximately five. Once again, patients could only receive the therapy if they consented and completed the diaries and questionnaires. A further advantage of the NADA protocol is that it requires no diagnostic skills and uses five standard fixed points in the ear; therefore, non-acupuncture practitioners can be trained relatively quickly to deliver the treatment. While the results of the two studies were being compiled and written up, two non-acupuncturists (one a reflexologist, the other a nurse) continued the service.

This approach for integrating research into the routine delivery of a therapy has led to the development of a new service to meet a high patient demand, delivered in an efficient manner to maximize patient benefit.

## Aromatherapy and relaxation

While the provision of aromatherapy massage in cancer centres and hospices is widespread, evidence for its effectiveness is still lacking. LJMC took part in a multi-centre randomized controlled trial, the initial aim of which was to compare aromatherapy massage and relaxation classes with a no-treatment control arm in patients with advanced cancer. (Patients randomized to the control arm could receive aromatherapy massage at the end of the study after a 6-week follow-up period.) However, the study was beset with problems in its initial design.

To increase the credibility of the results, the study had rigorous entry criteria, requiring patients to consent to a psychiatric interview to diagnose anxiety or mild–moderate depression. Only those patients with a definite diagnosis could then consent to be randomized. This dual-consent procedure deterred some patients from participating, especially as the usual service was running alongside the trial. At times, when the waiting list for aromatherapy massage was short, patients could gain access to immediate aromatherapy massage anyway and the relaxation classes were open to all on a drop-in basis without appointment. In addition, when patients were first screened for potential eligibility for the study, they often appeared anxious or depressed but by the time an appointment had been made for the diagnostic interview a few days later, this was no longer the case.

The study was initially open only to patients with advanced cancer. However, some health professionals felt it was unethical to carry out research on this group, so they either stopped making referrals altogether or ensured that their patients were referred direct to the service. For patients who self-referred, their first contact with the LJMC was often through volunteers, who were not always able to ascertain their disease stage and decide whether it was appropriate to mention the research study. These problems and others are discussed by Westcombe *et al.* (2003). Eventually, the study was opened to patients at any stage of disease and the randomization was simplified to aromatherapy versus control (or delayed aromatherapy).

Results from the study (Wilkinson *et al.* 2007) indicate that patients who received aromatherapy massage were significantly less distressed at 4 weeks post-treatment but a reduction in distress was also found in the control group and the difference between the groups was not significant. Patients in the aromatherapy massage group were also significantly less distressed immediately post-treatment compared to baseline and this difference was significantly larger than that in the control arm. One interpretation of these results is that the diagnostic interviews pre- and post-treatment were therapeutic in themselves. The Cavendish Centre in Sheffield has long recognized the value of their initial assessment interview and therefore take on extra staff to ensure the waiting list for this is never too long, although there may then be a wait for the recommended therapy (Peace and Manasse 2002).

Both the acupuncture and the aromatherapy studies demonstrate the need to ensure that research protocols are flexible and can adapt to accommodate changes in circumstances, without losing scientific integrity. Integrating research in the routine delivery of complementary therapies improves the credibility of the centre.

# References

Brumbaugh, A. G. 1994, *Transformation and Recovery: A Guide for the Design and Development of Acupuncture-based Chemical Dependency Treatment Programs*. Santa Barbara, Still Point.

Corner, J., Harewood, J., Maslin-Porthero, S. *et al.* 2006, A study of the use of complementary and alternative therapies among people undergoing cancer treatment. A quantitative and qualitative study. Available at: www.dh.gov.uk/publicationsandstatistics

de Valois, B., Young, T., Hunter, M., Lucey, R. & Maher, E. J. 2002, Using traditional acupuncture for hot flushes and night sweats in women taking Tamoxifen – a pilot study, *Focus on Alternative and Complementary Therapies (FACT)*, 2002, vol. **8**, no. 1, pp. 134–5.

de Valois, B., Young, T., Hunter, M. & Maher, E. J. 2003, Evaluating physical and emotional well-being in women using traditional acupuncture to manage tamoxifen side effects, *Focus on Alternative and Complementary Therapies (FACT)*, vol. **8**, no. 4, p. 492.

House of Lords, Science and Technology, Sixth Report 2000.

Howells, N. & Maher, E. J. 1998, Complementary therapists and cancer patient care: developing a regional network to promote co-operation, collaboration, education and patient choice, *European Journal of Cancer Care*, vol. **7**, pp. 129–34.

Kite, S. M., Maher, E. J., Anderson, K. *et al.* 1998, Development of an aromatherapy service at a cancer centre, *Palliative Medicine*, vol. **12**, pp. 171–80.

NICE Guidelines: Improving supportive and palliative care for adults with cancer. The Manual. 2004 (available at: www.nice.org.uk).

Peace, G. & Manasse, A. 2002, The Cavendish Centre for integrated cancer care: assessment of patients needs and responses, *Complementary Therapies in Medicine*, vol. **10**, pp. 33–41.

Westcombe, A. M., Gambles, M. A., Young, T. *et al.* 2003, Learning the hard way! Setting up an RCT of aromatherapy massage for patients with cancer, *Palliative Medicine*, vol. **17**, pp. 300–7.

Wilkinson, S. M., Love, S. B., Westcombe, A. M. *et al.* 2007, Effectiveness of aromatherapy massage in the management of anxiety and depression in patients with cancer: a randomised controlled trial, *Journal of Clinical Oncology*, vol. **25**, pp. 532–9.

Chapter 4

# The hospice setting

Nigel Hartley

## Summary

Complementary therapy services have been developed in many hospices over the last 20 years. More recently, questions have been raised regarding which therapy or therapies should be used alongside orthodox medical treatment and who should be administering them. Training, supervision, and proof of the efficacy of such therapies are becoming paramount as many hospices and specialist palliative care units take the opportunity to reformulate complementary therapies within their service provision plans. In this chapter, the development and evaluation of the professional service provided by nurse therapists at St. Christopher's Hospice is described.

## Introduction

'I had a patient today and she said something really, really nice: "within this time with you… I found me"'. Extract from therapist interview quoted by Bell and Atkins (2006)

St. Christopher's Hospice in the UK is credited as the 'birthplace of the modern hospice movement…' (Small 2003). Opened in 1967, it has grown into a large community resource providing care for patients living with a variety of terminal illnesses and life-threatening conditions and for their carers. This care is underpinned by an international education programme for healthcare professionals and a commitment to 'public education' for those who live within the local community. Research and evaluation into the care provided has been paramount from the outset and the hospice works in partnership with many higher educational establishments to use existing research paradigms and develop new ones, which are appropriate and ethical to end-of-life care.

Complementary therapies have been available to patients free of charge at St. Christopher's for a number of years but only in the past 2 years has the formalization of what is offered become central to the establishment. This has meant examining the background and qualification of practitioners, adequate supervision and support, integration into patients' care packages, an expanding educational role, and building up research evidence. The aim of this chapter is to examine how and why this formalization of the complementary therapy service has come about, highlight the risks and rewards of such a venture, share some findings of a recent qualitative research study, and articulate some very real challenges for the future.

## How do hospices define complementary therapies?

The terms 'complementary' and 'alternative' provide material for much debate in healthcare, particularly in specialist palliative care. There are many definitions of 'complementary therapies'. Most of them mention that this range of treatments is used alongside or mixed together with orthodox medical treatment. This implies a distinction from 'alternative' therapies, which are often the same types of therapies also known as 'complementary' but being used instead of orthodox medicine. Hospices attach prime importance to patients' choice of treatment and would rarely condone any therapy as 'alternative' to conventional medical treatment; rather, these therapies would be part of a treatment programme that uses conventional methods also.

Which specific therapies should be provided as part of a care package for terminally ill patients is also a source of debate. This is partly due to the lack of evidence available to support many of the complementary therapies. Most hospices consider 'patient choice' as central and most provide some or all of the so-called core touch therapies: massage, aromatherapy massage, and reflexology. Other therapies that have come to be used widely in recent years include psychologically based ones such as hypnotherapy, relaxation, and stress management. All these interventions are available at St. Christopher's because they are the therapies that have the most proof of efficacy from studies undertaken in various parts of the UK. At St. Christopher's, these therapies are regulated through a growing body of research and evaluation.

The lack of regulation of complementary therapies in UK has caused some problems when attempts were made to integrate them into healthcare services; however, the publication of the National Guidelines for the Use of Complementary Therapies in Supportive and Palliative Care (Tavares 2003) has provided useful guidance on training, therapy provision, support, supervision, and efficacy. This publication has stimulated many healthcare establishments to redefine or reorganize their therapy services and it is an important step in the development of these services for the future.

## Who should deliver complementary therapies in specialist palliative care?

The hospice movement has used volunteers from the outset; people have volunteered their time in various ways, mainly in a supportive role to paid staff in their work with patients. Specialist palliative day care services depend on volunteers to support the social context of the work through tasks such as providing refreshments and serving lunch. Complementary therapies within hospices have often grown up initially within day care centres and have traditionally been provided by volunteers with some training in complementary therapy techniques such as massage and relaxation. In the early years of St. Christopher's, volunteer nurses and physiotherapists provided support for the work. This type of volunteering has diminished over the years due to the growing, essential regulative aspects of various healthcare professions. It appears that complementary therapies are also currently moving in the same direction and if this is the case, the days of volunteers providing complementary therapies must be drawing to a close. The question of who should be providing complementary therapies within specialist palliative care has currently attracted considerable attention and has been debated from various angles. The current view point at St. Christopher's is that since it is involved in delivering specialist palliative care, all services should be of high standard, provided by professionals with experience, knowledge, and wisdom (Trevalyn and Booth 1994). Therefore, at St. Christopher's, service is now provided by nurse therapists—specialist palliative care nurses who are also qualified to practise complementary therapies.

These nurse therapists are able not only to deliver quality complementary therapy treatments but also to work closely with the medical team in terms of pain and symptom management. We find that complementary therapists have access to patient's bodies in a way that even medical practitioners sometimes do not; for example, patients readily remove their clothes for massage, so that therapists may witness severe disfigurement due to illness or treatment and notice changes that are important to pass on to the medical team. Therefore, it appears sensible that complementary therapists also be experienced healthcare professionals because they are dealing with complex specialist healthcare issues. This is not to say that volunteers may not have a role to play in the delivery of complementary therapies within hospices—what that role is needs careful consideration.

## How should complementary therapists be trained, supported, and supervised?

### How should people be trained to provide complementary therapies within specialist healthcare settings?

There are many ways to train as a complementary therapist in the UK, particularly in massage. These range from weekend courses to full-blown courses at the diploma and degree levels. In specialist healthcare settings, it could be argued that degree-level training should be treated as the benchmark against which practice and efficacy can be measured.

## Who should provide support for and supervise complementary therapists working in healthcare?

Volunteer complementary therapists are managed by different people, depending on the hospice they work in. These range from volunteer co-ordinators, often with no experience in complementary therapies, to nurses and managers from various departments. Experience shows that when setting up a volunteer complementary therapy service in a hospice, the assistance of a full-time designated healthcare professional is necessary to manage the service in terms of providing adequate training, support and supervision, and overseeing research and evaluation projects. Some managers offer one-to-one or group supervision, with some hospices engaging professionals outside of the hospice staff to play the role of a facilitator.

## How should effective research and evaluation procedures be identified and developed?

Lack of proof of efficacy of complementary therapies is an ongoing concern. Involving volunteers in research and evaluation may be difficult because they have only limited time and usually prefer to spend it on activities that involve direct contact with the people they are helping to support. Also, there may be problems regarding lack of experience and an unwillingness to allow scrutiny of their work. Understanding the work in the context of the hospice multi-professional team can be complex too, with volunteers often being unable to attend meetings because of the part-time nature of their work. Communication and management structures seldom include opportunities to involve volunteers in a professional sense. At St. Christopher's, we have used our contacts with local academic institutions to support our questions around the work, help identify suitable research paradigms, and work with the therapists to sustain enquiry into what they do.

## How do complementary therapists talk about their work?

Language provides us with a very real dilemma. When complementary therapists talk about their work, they do not always convey effective descriptions of what is actually involved. Administering complementary therapy is not the same as talking about it, and in turn, is not the same as researching its efficacy. Until complementary therapists find a common language that can define and explain their work, it will be difficult to integrate their treatments fully into healthcare practice, due to the misunderstandings and complications that can arise from talking about what goes on during sessions.

## Why use nurses to deliver complementary therapies?

By using nurses to deliver complementary therapies at St. Christopher's, we find that many of the preceding issues become irrelevant. When we set up a community complementary therapy service, many local family doctors (GPs) were anxious about complementary therapies being delivered within patient's homes. Once they realized that the therapists were also experienced specialist palliative care nurses, their fears were allayed. Right or wrong, this was the case, and enabled us to provide a service that was supported by community physicians. With regard to language, these nurses are experienced in talking to all kinds of health and social care professionals. Although explaining complementary therapies is complex for nurses too, we find that people are keener to listen and develop an understanding. Until the issues with regard to regulation and effective levels of complementary therapy training in the UK are resolved, with the need to prove their worth and provide safe practice, it seems sensible that nurses who are dually qualified as complementary therapists are the ones to take the cause further.

## The Hospice setting

In 2007, St. Christopher's Hospice celebrates its fortieth anniversary. Our local community of 1.8 million people is one of the most ethnically diverse populations in the UK. Over the 40 years, this has changed from a mainly white middle-class area into one that is more multi-faceted economically, socially, and politically. Due to this diversity, the needs of dying patients and their families in our community are many and varied and have changed over this time. In addition to those terminally ill due to various forms of cancer, we care for an increasing number of patients with end-stage non-malignant conditions such as motor neurone disease, AIDS, multiple sclerosis, heart failure, and renal failure. Caring for the elderly who are terminally ill is also a current focus and growing responsibility.

The 'hospice setting' is not just a building. At St. Christopher's, on any given day, we are caring for up to 600 patients and their families and carers. With 48 beds in our Inpatient Unit, 20 places a day in our Day Care Unit, and a limited outpatient clinic service, most of these users are looked after in their own homes. In addition to providing a complementary therapy service to patients, families, and carers on the hospice site, we have developed a community-based complementary therapy service during the last year; two of our therapists, both of whom previously practised as community nurse specialists, deliver this service to patients at the places where they live. One of the main benefits of their community nursing background has been the ability to discourse with other healthcare professionals in the community, particularly family doctors, and also their knowledge of diseases other than cancer. This busy and energetic service is the subject of an ongoing research project.

Support services for carers of dying patients have become central to the political agenda in the UK over the past couple of years. Hospices have always put the family, as well as the patient, as central to their philosophy. A current plan at St. Christopher's is to develop a complementary therapy service for carers to be delivered at the places where they live because constraints of time and money often prevent those engaged in full-time caring from accessing supportive services in any other way. Of carers who took part in the UK government's consultation 'Your Health, Your Care, Your Say', 79% reported that their health was worse due to caring, 58% presented with significant depression, 91% with stress and worry, and 50% with chronic backache (Department of Health 2006). Results from our completed research projects tell us that massage is a particularly useful therapy for alleviating depression, stress, and physical pain in patients who are terminally ill. Therefore, it seems sensible to examine this with reference to the needs of carers also.

## Practice, education, and research: a complementary therapy study for St. Christopher's Hospice

The birth of the hospice was based on the trinity of practice, education, and research. When developing complementary therapies, this still remains the case. If complementary therapies are to be accepted by the cross-section of specialist palliative care professionals working in hospices, we must enquire into their efficacy as rigorously and as effectively as possible.

In 2005, St. Christopher's embarked on a research study in partnership with Kingston University/St. George's University in London. Copies of the final report (Bell and Atkins 2006), from which most of the information in this section is taken, can be obtained from St Christopher's.

The aims of the study were:

◆ To investigate the views of patients, nurses, and therapists about the complementary therapies (specifically hypnotherapy, aromatherapy, massage, and reflexology) that are provided by St. Christopher's Hospice and the South East Cancer Help Centre (a local cancer drop-in centre that also provides complementary therapies)

- To provide the hospice with information and recommendations that could be used to inform decisions about the future provision of complementary therapies

Following an in-depth literature review, semi-structured interviews were conducted with three samples of people: staff who referred patients for complementary therapies, patients who received the therapies, and therapists who delivered them. Due to the nature of end-of-life care, recruitment of patients to the study was difficult. However, 54 patients were interviewed, which is a relatively high number compared to other studies. The profile of the patients who were interviewed reflected the general population of the hospice catchment area.

Recordings of the interviews were analyzed and themes emerged as follows:

- Positive effects of complementary therapy
- Adverse effects of complementary therapy
- The patients who gain most and least from complementary therapy
- Patients' relationships with the therapists
- Attitudes of doctors and nurses towards complementary therapy
- Complementary therapy not a cure
- Therapists' understanding of cancer

The final report draws together findings from the study as follows:

- Almost all the patients, therapists, and nurses who were interviewed expressed the view that the complementary therapies provided were complementary to orthodox medical treatment, rather than an alternative to it
- When patients talk about their conventional treatment... they... describe periods of great anxiety, things happening very rapidly, of pain, of discomfort, of not understanding what was happening to them and a loss of control... they perceive themselves being treated as objects rather than as people with feelings... patients' descriptions of complementary therapies... refer to their positive relationship with the therapists, of being able to talk and be listened to, about being recognized as people with a life beyond their cancer diagnosis
- A main theme identified from patient interviews was that complementary therapy occupies the space between being 'normal'—having an ordinary life, living at home, going to work, being well and 'abnormal'—having cancer, being in a hospice, being a patient
- It is very clear that all patients enjoyed the complementary therapy and a large majority (95%)—some of whom had been sceptical about complementary

therapy—believed that they had benefited … these benefits included increased relaxation and calmness, decreased anxiety, reduction in pain, improved feelings of well-being, positive impact on emotions, and improved sleep patterns

◆ Patients, therapists, and nurses said that the therapeutic techniques themselves provided the benefits experienced by the patients. However, they also suggested that some of the more interpersonal aspects such as the relationship with the therapist, touch, and communication were helpful. Some interviewees said that the relationship between the therapist and patient was even more important than the therapeutic techniques, while others suggested that it was of minimal importance

A number of recommendations were made following completion of the study and they include the following:

◆ …complementary therapy appears to reduce the symptoms associated with …illnesses, including anxiety, stress, and pain…we recommend that the hospice…continue with complementary therapy and consider ways in which complementary therapy might be extended and expanded

◆ …complementary therapy sessions are one-to-one with patients and often involve the patients divulging very personal and distressing information…. We recommend that the hospice review the support and supervision offered to therapists to ensure that quality assurance issues and staff welfare issues are addressed appropriately

## Conclusion

'…I have tried green tea and I didn't really like it at all and you know I'm sort of working out my thoughts about things you don't like because you want to make life as enjoyable as possible and if drinking green tea gives you say an extra six months but you don't enjoy it, well that's not really what life is about…' Extract from patient interview quoted by Bell and Atkins (2006).

At St. Christopher's Hospice Creative Living Centre, which provides creative and complementary resources to patients, families, and carers living with and caring for people with end-of-life disease both in the hospice building and in the local community, complementary therapies make up some of our most popular services. There is usually a waiting list and people are always wanting more. Despite the lack of evidence, the difficulties regarding who should be providing them, and issues regarding training, support, and supervision, people tell us that complementary therapies are important to them during the progression of their terminal disease.

Our experience tells us that for patients approaching death, issues of time are paramount and so they refuse to engage in activities that have little or no meaning or that are not enjoyable. The 'user's voice' has become more central to healthcare in the UK (Saunders 2003) with users' groups being set up to provide advice and guidance in a changing healthcare system. If we really take note of what patients are saying, complementary therapies are here to stay. Our responsibility is to educate users to make an informed choice, enable treatments to be safe through rigorous training and research, and to be open to, and to welcome, constructive criticism.

Integrating complementary therapies into the hospice setting is an ongoing objective.

## References

Bell, L. & Atkins, C. 2006, *Complementary therapies study for St. Christopher's Hospice – final report*. St. Christopher's Hospice, London.

Department of Health 2006, *Our health, our care, our say: a new direction for community services*. White Paper. Department of Health, London.

Saunders, C. 2003, In *Patient Participation in Palliative Care: A Voice for the Voiceless*, B. Monroe & D. Oliviere, ed. Oxford University Press, Oxford. pp. 3–8.

Small, N. 2003, In *Patient Participation in Palliative Care: A Voice for the Voiceless*, B. Monroe & D. Oliviere, ed. Oxford University Press, Oxford. pp. 9–22.

Tavares, M. 2003, *National guidelines for the use of complementary therapies in supportive and palliative care*. Prince of Wales's Foundation for Integrated Health, London.

Trevalyn, J. & Booth, B. 1994, *Complementary Medicine for Nurses, Midwives and Health Visitors*. Macmillan Press, London.

Chapter 5

# The work of an independent cancer help centre

Sara R Miller and Ruth Sewell

## Summary

As the UK's leading holistic cancer charity, Penny Brohn Cancer Care (formerly the Bristol Cancer Help Centre) has pioneered the *Bristol Approach* to care for people diagnosed with cancer and those close to them. This approach works alongside mainstream cancer treatment, providing a combination of physical, emotional, and spiritual support, using complementary therapies and self-help techniques including practical advice on nutrition.

## Introduction

Penny Brohn Cancer Care, situated close to the city of Bristol, was founded in 1980 by Penny Brohn, a woman diagnosed with breast cancer, and her friend Pat Pilkington. The Bristol Approach is the result of many years' clinical experience. The emphasis is on supporting people/patients to enjoy the benefits of receiving complementary therapies while also helping them learn to use self-help approaches. Practical advice is given on complementary approaches that can help relieve cancer-related symptoms, and on the management of treatment side effects, along with nutritional recommendations to help people deal with problems at any time from diagnosis onwards. The programme is also designed to be accessible to family members or friends who are supporting the person with cancer. The Bristol Approach combined with medical treatment provides a model of integrative whole-person care starting from the time of diagnosis, continuing through treatment, into post-cancer rehabilitation and on-going well-being, and during the palliative phase of the illness.

Scientific evidence continues to support the importance of an integrative approach to cancer and its treatment. For over two decades, there has been increasing research evidence indicating important links between illness, emotional well-being, thoughts, and the communication between these factors influencing the body's response. Psychoneuroimmunology (PNI) is the study of connections between the mind, nervous system, and immune system. This is becoming increasingly relevant to the therapeutic approaches utilized in the Bristol Approach.

The psycho-immunology of cancer (Lewis *et al.* 2002) provides an in-depth review of the evidence to date of the way in which the mind may influence the body in cancer and in the Preface, the authors note:

> 'When the first edition of this book came out in 1994, the psycho-immunology of cancer was still emerging as a topic for serious scientific study. Now less than ten years later, there is a huge academic literature about the relationships between psychological variables, the immune system and cancer growth, accompanied by a lively popular interest'.

## Qualitative studies of the Bristol Approach

A qualitative research study published by the Charity (then known as the Bristol Cancer Help Centre) highlighted the importance of providing complementary supportive care for people throughout their cancer journey and its particular importance at key points of vulnerability (Turton and Cooke 2000). In addition, the Measure Yourself Concerns and Well-being (MYCaW) questionnaire was developed to measure the concerns of service users (Paterson and Britten 2000). In 2005, the MYCaW questionnaire was administered to 189 people before and after they attended the Bristol Approach 2-day and Bristol Retreat 5-day residential courses and the data collated (Paterson *et al.* 2007). On arrival, people were asked to write down '*One or two concerns or problems which you would most like us to help you with*'. Examples of typical concerns ranged from needing nutritional advice, pain management or self-help techniques, to the effects of cancer on family and other relationships and work, and maintaining quality of life. These concerns were rated in severity from 0 '*Not bothering me at all*' to 6 '*Bothers me greatly*'. After their visit to the centre, people were asked to re-score their concerns. Results show a statistically significant improvement (Fig. 5.1).

Ongoing evaluation is being undertaken in order to ensure that the programme accurately matches, and meets, the needs of those who use the services.

## Components of the Bristol Approach

The Bristol Approach combines complementary therapies and stress-reducing self-help techniques, along with providing emotional support and practical advice on healthy eating and lifestyle. Interventions on offer include:

- ◆ *Group sessions* for sharing, mutual support, and learning; to help reduce fear and isolation and improve the quality of life; and to aid in recovery or preparation for death

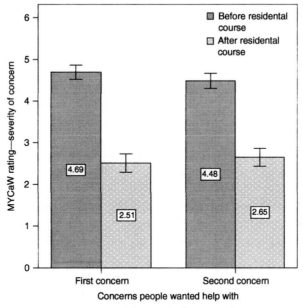

**Figure 5.1** Patients' concern ratings before and after attending course.

- *Meditation and healing* to address spiritual aspects, promote peace of mind, and reduce fear and anxiety
- *Relaxation and imagery techniques* to help people regain a sense of control over their situation, restore a sense of meaning and purpose in their lives, and give support during treatment
- *Counselling and psychotherapy* to help people address emotional issues, come to terms with changes in their lives, and look forward
- *Nutritional advice*, including guidelines on healthy food choices and the use of supplements and herbs, where appropriate, to support the body in its self-healing processes, improve health and well-being, and support the immune system
- *Touch therapies* such as massage and shiatsu to reduce anxiety, reduce pain, promote relaxation, and enhance energy levels
- *Creative therapies*, such as art and music therapy, for helping people to express feelings that they may not be able to articulate verbally
- *Gentle exercises* to improve oxygenation and circulation
- *Integrative medical sessions* that act as a bridge between the worlds of mainstream and complementary medicine, supporting the persons in taking

charge of their situation and thereby helping them prepare for, cope with, and benefit more from medical treatment.

The Bristol Approach is thought to be the only programme of its kind in the UK and is among the few in the world to comprehensively address all these different components as part of a coherent, integrative therapeutic strategy.

## Accessing the Bristol Approach

Ways of accessing the Bristol Approach range from the helpline, library, information and retail services, to attending single-day courses and/or residential courses.

Those living close to the centre are able to attend the community support programme Cancerpoint, which offers a range of one-to-one appointments including massage, shiatsu, reflexology, healing, acupuncture, and psychotherapy, with additional longer courses in art therapy and creative writing, as well as weekly support groups. Outreach programmes designed for local National Health Service Primary Health Care and local communities are also delivered within the Cancerpoint programme. The Bristol Approach is also offered through single-day courses and residential courses that offer an in-depth opportunity to experience the approach as presented by experienced teams of doctors, psychotherapists, nurses, and complementary therapists.

### Helpline

The initial point of contact for many people is the National Telephone Helpline. This service offers information on the Bristol Approach and guidance in finding qualified complementary therapists, support groups, and complementary therapy support services in the caller's local area. Helpline volunteers are also trained in listening and responding skills to support callers, whatever their reason for contacting the Charity. In 2005, there were over 10,000 enquiries to the telephone and email services. The email service appears to have encouraged more men to make contact, and is proving convenient for people from overseas.

### Starter pack

The self-help starter pack includes a DVD and a CD. The DVD provides a detailed overview of the various therapies and courses offered and an introduction to the Bristol Approach to complementary cancer care. It helps people to see the various ways in which they can actively influence their health and well-being—including healthy eating, relaxation, meditation, psychotherapy, and using complementary therapies. This is key after diagnosis, when people often feel they have 'lost control'. Learning how to relax, meditate, or prepare healthy food may seem simple but it helps to give back this sense of control; people become involved in promoting their own health rather than feeling impotent to affect change.

The CD includes examples of simple relaxation, meditation, and imagery exercises, each one introducing and guiding the listener towards integrating such self-help approaches into their daily lives. In addition, the self-help starter pack gives information on the Bristol Approach to healthy eating and vitamin and dietary supplement guidelines.

## Cancerpoint

Cancerpoint provides individual sessions in a range of complementary therapies, self-help techniques, and psychotherapy. This has proved to be an immensely popular facility, with many people using Cancerpoint alone, particularly as a support during treatment, and others attending as a follow on from a single-day or residential course. In addition to the facilities and programme of therapies within the Charity's building, programmes and courses on techniques such as relaxation have been successfully implemented into a variety of other settings in Bristol and beyond. The Charity is also able to provide reading and audio-visual resources within the library along with public access to CanHelpNow, a shop facility and mail order service that also supplies vitamin and dietary supplements.

## Single-day courses

Single-day courses, offered regularly throughout the year, provide access to individual elements of the programme, for example:

- Relaxation exercises and Breathwork
- Meditation and imagery
- Healthy eating and nutrition for people living with cancer

## Half-day events

Half-day events, such as the 'Taste of the Bristol Approach' course, introduce the principles of the programme and the variety of services that can help people gain a greater awareness of what types of therapies and/or support they might want to access.

## Residential courses

Residential courses form a major part of the service, attracting participants both from the UK and overseas. The courses run every week throughout the year, with shorter follow-up courses being offered regularly. Although these courses levy a fee, they are subsidized by the Charity, along with additional packages to support those on low income to ensure full access.

These residential courses offer 12 places to individuals over the age of 18 years. They are suitable for people at all stages of their cancer experience, ranging from diagnosis, during and following treatment, into remission, and following any recurrence of disease. Participants should be well enough to stay in hotel-type accommodation because the Charity is unable to provide medical or nursing care. Supporters are seen as having equal importance, although with different needs, and therefore are offered essentially the same programme with some additional input to help them identify their own needs while seeking to effectively support the person with cancer. The supporter can be a spouse, an adult child, a sibling, a parent, or a friend.

The residential courses stand out as providing in-depth opportunities for participants to reflect on their total situation and so have the potential to review the things that are important to them and their quality of life and well-being. For many, this is a life-enhancing and life-changing experience.

There are residential courses lasting 2 days and 5 days. *Introduction to the Bristol Approach* is a 2-day course providing a detailed overview of the principles underpinning the therapeutic approaches, along with individual guidance on how the participants can individualize their experiences after attending. The *Bristol Retreat* is a 5-day course that not only informs participants of the underpinning principles and provides individual guidance but also gives them more time to reflect and come to terms with their illness, with additional support from the others present. During the 5-day retreat, participants also receive body therapies such as shiatsu and massage, healing, music therapy, art therapy, and focused time for learning and perfecting self-help techniques of relaxation, meditation, and imagery. Course members have the chance to review their situation and gain support from the team of therapists and other participants. This can help them to renew their self-help practices and review their lifestyle choices and enable them to make any necessary changes to improve their quality of life and levels of health and well-being.

A warm welcome and a relaxing evening set the scene for the residential courses. Close bonds of friendship can form, especially during the 5-day retreat course, and serve as lasting sources of support. Ideally, it is recommended to attend the 2-day Bristol Approach course first and then to enhance the experience at a later date with the 5-day Bristol Retreat course. Since this is not always practical, some participants decide to start by attending the retreat. There may be a wide range of experiences of an integrated approach among those attending, with some for whom the Bristol Approach is a totally new concept and others who may have been practising aspects of it for many years.

Participants on a course may also be at very different stages of disease process. All these varying aspects are brought together by the therapy team to create a rich and cohesive group experience for the participants.

Following attendance on a course, participants are encouraged and supported in developing a self-care programme to put into action at home. This may include, for example, seeking groups and centres in their local area for support in continuing their self-help practice. The Charity also provides a range of follow-up support, including free phone-in nutritional therapy and doctor phone-in services, accessible to all who have attended a residential course. For those who live close to the Charity, individual appointments with therapists and doctors are available through Cancerpoint.

It is easy for us to describe the benefits of our residential courses; however, what really matters is the experience of those who attend. One course participant, Mac Jeffery, gives the following account:

'The diagnosis of choroidal melanoma was a terrible shock. I had a large tumour, 9 mm, in my right eye. I was offered either plaque radiotherapy or enucleation and, after a disturbed week, I chose enucleation. The medical treatment and care I received was excellent. But I was exhausted, scared, distressed and angry.

I knew if I was to support my medical treatment and build my immune system to prevent the reoccurrence of cancer, I needed to find out what I could do to help myself, so I attended a two day residential course at the Bristol Cancer Help Centre. I went holding on to my feelings, tensions and confusion but there I learnt to "let go" of them.

Through counselling and art therapy I was able to express my fears, anger and distress with people who I could trust and who accepted me. I could share my experience of cancer with others on the course and listen to their stories. I wasn't alone.

I "let go" of the tensions in my body learning to deeply relax using guided imagery and visualizations. I perfected my visualization to help in my fight against cancer. I used a dragon image, as this clearly represented the anger I was feeling. I imagined my dragon patrolling through my body, directing its flaming breath on cancer cells and burning them up. I then added a flock of white doves to clear up the remains of the cancer cells.

I "let go" of my assumptions about diet and complementary therapies. The recommended cancer diet wasn't raw and bland but full of taste, colour, and nutrition. I learnt about new foods and a number of recipes, which inspired my cooking. I went with an open mind to Spiritual Healing and it was a wonderful and profound experience.

The Bristol Approach enabled me to regain control over my health and well-being. It proved to be the catalyst for many changes in my life. There were things that I could do to help my body, mind and spirit and now was the time to do them!'

## The team

The strength and essence of the Charity's approach lies in the commitment to work mindfully within a democratic and supportive organization. Every individual, whether he/she is in the administration, fund-raising, or therapy part of the team, joins in the blended and co-operative approach to the work that seeks to move as a whole.

The therapy team responsible for residential courses includes doctors specializing in integrative medicine, transpersonal psychotherapists, nurse therapists, nutritional therapists, healers, art therapists, massage therapists, shiatsu practitioners, and music therapists, supported by course co-ordinators and night assistants. The team is remarkable in its cohesiveness, given that any combination of therapists may be working together on a course. This may be explained by the unity of working for a common aim but is undoubtedly enhanced by the underlying spiritual foundation of Penny Brohn Cancer Care. Non-denominational, the Charity supports a belief that we each have a spirit and that it is the state of our spirit that determines how we cope with life's challenges.

When life loses its meaning, the person may lose the will to live. Finding a new reason to live when dreams have been shattered restores purpose, renews hope, and raises self-esteem. There is always something worth hoping for: a full recovery, the absence of recurrence, time to fulfil dreams, to live well even in the presence of life-threatening or life-reducing illness, and, ultimately, hope for a peaceful and good death. The discovery of meaning and of hope sustains the individual through the experience of cancer.

Developing a creative outlet, through art for example, often awakens new potential and becomes a source of fulfilment. Therapists working at the centre, whatever their discipline, hold in their consciousness the potential for wholeness for each person. This is spiritual work, which sustains both the therapist, in the face of pain and suffering, and the client. It enables both to be with uncomfortable feelings and acknowledge them without the need to placate or negate them. This in itself can be a deeply healing experience.

Handover meetings provide continuity of care, always utilizing a holistic view of participants' needs. Team members have the support of supervision, peer group and therapy team meetings, regular evaluations, and annual appraisals along with meeting with the head of therapy at any time over specific issues or difficulties. A core group, consisting of clinical director, head of therapy, the therapy course manager, and senior members of the team representing each discipline, meets monthly to support and develop all aspects of the programme, ensuring its smooth operation. This has proved to be an effective method of management.

## The doctors

The doctors work in an integrative way, bringing together mainstream medical knowledge with the principles of PNI and other modalities that serve to look at the person as a whole—body, mind, emotions, and spirit. The aim is to restore 'wholeness', with emphasis on health and healing rather than primarily on disease and treatment.

The work of the Charity complements and enhances the medical care for those receiving, or having received, treatment for cancer. To this end, the doctors can:

- Interpret medical 'jargon'
- Explain treatment modalities
- Recommend complementary symptom control
- Support the person with difficult treatment choices
- Provide support, empowerment, and a truly person-centred experience of the doctor–patient relationship
- Evaluate stress and lifestyle, including exercise, support, and overall state of well-being
- Teach the principles of PNI

Emphasis is placed on gradual change, appropriate to the individual's capacity and energy levels, allowing new habits to form at a natural pace. Low energy levels, as a result of treatments or of the cancer itself, can lead to low self-esteem, reduced pain tolerance, and a lack of motivation. To suggest major life changes at this point could simply compound the exhaustion and increase hopelessness, rather than helping.

As a part of energy enhancement, good-quality balanced information is discussed and individual recommendations made regarding the dietary vitamins, minerals, and supplements that have been shown to be of benefit to people with a cancer diagnosis. The Charity has put together its own Bristol Pack of recommended supplements, with research-based policies on their use during chemotherapy and radiotherapy. The use of supplements during chemotherapy is subject to major controversy, with strong arguments both for and against their use (Block 2004). The senior doctor regularly checks research papers and consults with peers in order to keep abreast of current research and thinking on nutritional supplements.

## Education for healthcare professionals and complementary therapists

Education is a mainstay of the Charity and a variety of courses are offered, some of them linked with university and academic centres. Upwards of 500 places a year for health professionals and complementary therapists provide in-depth courses on the Bristol Approach and related subjects such as PNI, transpersonal psychotherapy, and holistic models of care for those affected by cancer. A unique educational opportunity for complementary therapists is found in the Certificate of Working with People with Cancer, which can also be taken as an academically accredited course. Other accredited courses designed for healthcare professionals are offered, highlighting the integrative approach to complementary therapies in current healthcare practices and in cancer care. Programmes are held throughout the year and attract both national and international delegates. These educational programmes are receiving greater national recognition in providing an integrative approach to cancer care and its educational responsibilities, as illustrated through the following quote from Professor Mike Richards, National Cancer Director, UK, in 2005:

> 'I applaud the work Bristol Cancer Help Centre is doing through its training programme for health professionals and complementary therapists'.

## Conclusion

Integrated cancer care is evolving as an evidence-based approach to caring, supporting, and long-term management for those individuals affected by cancer. This model represents a unified form of mainstream treatment, psychological and supportive care, and complementary therapies. The aim is to enhance the efficacy of treatment, improve symptom control, and alleviate suffering. An integrated approach emphasizes the importance of the individual, encouraging and enabling them to be involved in their treatment and beyond. This can increase their perception of control, while affording them greater insight into ways of taking responsibility for enhancing their quality of life. Professor Karol Sikora has described the Bristol Approach as '*the gold standard for complementary care in cancer*'.

## References

Block, K. 2004, Antioxidants and cancer therapy; furthering the debate, *Integrative Cancer Therapies* vol. 3, no. 4, pp. 342–8.

Lewis, C. E., O'Brien, R. M., Barraclough, J. (eds) 2002, *The Psycho-immunology of Cancer*, Oxford University Press, Oxford.

Paterson, C. & Britten, N. 2000, In pursuit of patient-centred outcomes: a qualitative evaluation of the 'Measure Yourself Medical Outcome Profile', *Journal of Health Services Research Policy* vol. 5, no. 1, pp. 27–36.

Paterson, C., Thomas, K., Manasse, A., Cooke, H., Peace, G. 2007, Measure Yourself Concerns and Well-being (MYCaW) questionnaire for evaluating outcome in cancer supportive care that includes complementary therapies. *Complementary therapies in medicine*, vol. 15, pp. 38–45.

Turton, P. & Cooke, H. 2000, Meeting the needs of people with cancer for support and self-management, *Complementary Therapies in Nursing and Midwifery*, vol. 6, pp. 130–7.

## Website

www.pennybrohncancercare.org

Chapter 6

# Childhood cancer

Elena J Ladas and Kara M Kelly

## Summary

Many parents of children and adolescents with cancer investigate complementary/alternative medicine (CAM) to help manage the side effects associated with conventional medications and augment their efficacy and to help cope with the diagnosis. Surveys have found that up to 84% of children with cancer use CAM (Kelly 2004), mostly in conjunction with conventional therapies rather than in lieu of those therapies. Parents pursue CAM to ensure that they have 'left no stone unturned' and feel they are doing all they can to help their child fight cancer or to support their child during cancer therapy. The high prevalence of CAM use has also brought attention to the potential for adverse interactions with conventional therapy, particularly when biological therapies (herbal or nutrition supplements) are used in combination with conventional agents. Although great strides have recently been made in elucidating the safety and efficacy of several CAM therapies, there is still a paucity of data regarding the use of CAM in combination with conventional therapy among children with cancer.

## Considerations regarding CAM for children with cancer

There are several unique factors either supporting or discouraging the use of CAM in children with cancer. Cancer in children is for the most part quite different from that in adults. The common childhood tumours are more sensitive to chemotherapy than are most adult carcinomas, such that today nearly 75% of children can expect to be cured. For some cancers such as Hodgkin lymphoma, non-Hodgkin lymphoma, Wilms' tumour, and germ cell tumours, the cure rate is more than 90%. Children tend to tolerate chemotherapy better as they are less likely to have co-morbid conditions. Therefore, it is imperative to avoid CAM therapies that may interfere with conventional therapies or to delay their use. In addition, there is significantly greater participation in clinical trials among children with cancer as compared with adults.

Therefore, concomitant use of any CAM therapy must be recorded so that any potential interactions can be carefully monitored.

There are many aspects of childhood cancer therapy where CAM may play a useful role. Practitioners are challenged with the need to support physical and intellectual growth. School, extra-curricular activities, and routine play dates can be abruptly interrupted with the diagnosis of cancer. A multidisciplinary approach is applied to help the child maintain some sense of normalcy while receiving treatment. This team approach typically includes physicians, child life specialists, nutritionists, psychologists, social workers, and nurses. As members of the multidisciplinary team, CAM practitioners focus on interventions to minimize pain and suffering and to provide practical, emotional, and physical support. CAM interventions, which are family-centred and child-focused, may be delivered in the inpatient or outpatient setting or at home. The decision to include CAM should be based on the evidence available: therapies that require a tremendous burden with unproven benefit or create obstacles for the child to adhere to the recommended therapy should be avoided.

CAM therapies may be a good resource for children whose illnesses or conventional treatments involve an extended period of stay in the hospital, such as those with newly diagnosed acute lymphoblastic leukaemia (ALL), those undergoing stem cell transplants, and those terminally ill. These children often become fatigued and have reduced muscle tone. CAM interventions such as yoga, karate, and massage can help maintain movement, muscle tone, and strength. Massage or reflexology can ease muscle pain and help motivate the child to adhere to exercise protocols.

The form of CAM and its appropriateness for the developmental age and planned conventional treatment of the child must be considered a priori. Conventional treatments associated with difficulty in swallowing, severe mouth sores, nausea and vomiting, or the use of nutrition support are likely to impact adherence to rigorous dietary changes or biologic CAM remedies. Children with fear of needles may have added anxiety with the use of acupuncture; acupressure or massage may be more appropriate options in such cases. Children may also have a fear of strangers and may assume that all healthcare providers will induce unintentional pain. Introducing the child to the CAM practitioners first with the help of child life specialists and the psychosocial team and then starting with the relatively non-invasive CAM modalities of reflexology, energy therapies, or aromatherapy may be more effective.

Conventional treatment regimens for cancer in children often take longer than those for adults. Some treatment plans for ALL include therapy for up to 3 consecutive years. This longer duration may motivate parents to search for more comprehensive approaches to the management of side effects or to investigate CAM therapies that may minimize the long-term effects of cancer therapy. On the other hand, CAM therapies that require numerous patient visits or require radical lifestyle modification may be unreasonable, given the demands of conventional treatment regimens.

Children may also need more explanation about CAM than do adults. A thorough discussion of the therapy and its demonstration may aid the child's decision to use CAM. Children are easily influenced by peers; therefore, observing a session on another patient, parent, or sibling may be beneficial. This is particularly true for younger patients who may not have the language skills to articulate their fears, yet have strong imaginations to understand concepts such as energy fields, guided imagery, and meditation.

The child's and the family's lifestyle, cultural and religious practices, as well as the child's diagnosis and planned conventional treatment regimen must be considered when advising patients on the use of CAM. These therapies may help to improve quality of life and may be associated with symptomatic benefit across the continuum of treatment for childhood cancer.

## Selected CAM therapies

### Acupuncture/acupressure

Acupuncture is the most thoroughly researched of traditional Chinese medicine (TCM) practices (Vickers *et al.* 2004). Acupuncture is generally accepted by children over the age of 6 years (Barnes and Berde 2000; Kemper *et al.* 2006; Reindl *et al.* 2006) and can help treat many of the symptoms experienced by children undergoing treatment for cancer, such as nausea and vomiting, pain, anxiety, insomnia, and fatigue (Ladas *et al.* 2006). Although data on acupuncture specifically in children with cancer is limited, two studies found that it was feasible (Reindl *et al.* 2006; Taromina *et al.* 2006).

An acupuncturist can readily treat multiple meridians in a single session, thereby helping with more than one condition at the same time. In order to sustain the effects of the treatment, the practitioner may provide the patient with press seeds or instruction on self-acupressure. This may be particularly effective for those at risk for delayed nausea, constipation, or neuropathy.

Acupuncture may be used with children of any age; however, special consideration must be given to those of certain age groups. Administration of acupuncture treatment to infants and toddlers often requires less rigorous techniques. The acupuncturist can stimulate the deficient/excess point for a few seconds, taking care not to retain the needles in the skin. This will reduce the risks of needle breakage or bacterial translocation associated with rapid movements by the patient. The use of fewer and smaller gauge needles, needle insertion with a guide tube, and shortened treatment duration will be more effective with children.

Children may be hesitant to receive acupuncture because it is not provided within the scope of conventional medicine or because it involves the application of needles. Discussion and demonstrations on a sibling, friend, or parent may help. Educating the medical staff on the acupuncture technique will also be useful.

## Case 1

An 11-year-old male was undergoing chemotherapy and beginning radiation therapy prior to resection of a synovial sarcoma in the left jaw region when treatment with acupuncture began.

The patient exhibited signs and symptoms of *qi* and *yin* deficiency associated with consecutive treatments of chemotherapy and radiation. Acupuncture points were selected to protect and tonify the patient's *qi* and *yin* (conception vessel 12, stomach 36, stomach 44, large intestine 4, 10, 11), stimulate the immune system (spleen 6, kidney 3 and 6), and alleviate local pain (stomach 6 and 7 and small intestine 18 and 19). These points were stimulated to decrease the possibility of delays in therapy, to boost the immune system, to tonify and protect the *qi* and *yin*, and for harmonization of the organs responsible for the production of *qi* and blood.

The patient received acupuncture, up to two treatments per week, prior to the surgical intervention. According to patient reports and the subjective findings by the acupuncturist at each session, a treatment principle, diagnosis, and protocol were developed and implemented. The acupuncture points selected varied between sessions, although certain points—anti-nausea (stomach 36 and pericardium 6) and immune-support (kidney 3 and 6)—were needled each time.

Prior to surgery, the primary objective was to protect the patient from the side effects of chemotherapy and radiation while supporting his overall constitution to promote well-being. During this time, the patient's reported symptoms included thickening of saliva and dry mouth, anxiety, and fatigue. The combination of the presence of the tumour and the radiation treatment created toxic heat that dried up the local fluids in the mouth, throat, and body. The main treatment principle was to clear toxic heat and regulate the organs through the stimulation of local and distal points along the affected channel, stomach and small intestine channel, and points that regulate the stomach organ. The patient was asked to suck a piece of candy throughout the acupuncture session to stimulate saliva production (Johnstone *et al.* 2002). After each treatment, the patient reported improvements in production of saliva.

Following surgery, the patient reported an inability to open his jaw and swelling in the local area of the tumour. Weekly acupuncture focused on relieving muscle spasms through local and distal points along the affected channels and included electroacupuncture, the use of microamperage for tissue repair in the local area. The patient was asked to insert tongue depressors in his mouth before and during the sessions to assist in loosening the jaw muscles and to gauge the effect of the treatment. He showed improvement during and immediately following treatment and reported that acupuncture made him 'feel better' each time. He reported little or no nausea and his energy and appetite improved following each treatment. There was also a reduction in allergy symptoms and feelings of increased relaxation. He has had a sustained resolution of xerostomia symptoms since the conclusion of treatment.

## Massage/reflexology

Massage is the systematic manipulation of soft tissues in the body (Ahles *et al.* 1999) and is one of the most widely used and accepted CAM therapies in children (Loman 2006), often being used to assist with pain management, reduce stress and anxiety, and support immune function. Studies have also reported that massage can reduce heart rate and diastolic blood pressure, reduce constipation, and improve the quality of life. Massage has been found to be an effective adjuvant therapy for individuals undergoing bone marrow transplant, with few reports of adverse effects and little possibility of interactions with therapy (Ahles *et al.* 1999).

Massage is generally considered safe for infants and children (Beachy 2003) and has the added benefit of being easily taught to parents, thereby the benefits can be extended outside the hospital setting. Massage provides parents with a non-invasive, comforting therapy to administer to their child, helping them feel they are playing a prominent role in their child's care. Massage is an ideal therapy to help manage pain after central venous catheter placement, biopsies, or lumbar punctures.

There are no known reported adverse effects in children when massage is provided by a licensed therapist. Practitioners should avoid areas of skin rupture, radiation burns, or other skin irritation. Massage should not be administered directly over a solid tumour and the practitioner should avoid the area in which a central venous catheter has been placed.

Reflexology is a form of massage that works through the stimulation of energy points on the feet or hands to bring homeostasis to the body and can be used during any part of the child's disease and healing process. Reflexology can readily be provided to infants and children and it helps to relieve side effects of cancer therapy. Because it requires minimal body contact, reflexology is an ideal therapy to introduce children to CAM. Even the most apprehensive child will often consent to their hands or feet being massaged.

---

### Case 2

A 3-year-old boy with stage-III Wilms' tumour was undergoing chemotherapy. While the child was at home, his mother observed that the boy had developed a shuffling gait with frequent falling episodes and had difficulty in maintaining balance. CAM consultation was requested. At the first meeting, the child was hesitant to meet any new practitioners or to allow them to touch him. The first visit consisted of discussion about massage/reflexology with the patient and demonstrations on his mother. After the second visit, the patient allowed the massage therapist to give leg massage and foot reflexology. The therapist began with reflexology by gently taking his foot and applying cream. The patient cried out 'Hey, that doesn't hurt'. He promptly extended his other foot for the same procedure. He continued receiving reflexology and leg massage. The parent was instructed on a range of movement exercises for the foot, including resistance exercises with the ankle. The child viewed the procedures as a game. After a few sessions, he began requesting massage on his right hand and arm; however, he would not consent to his left hand, arm, and shoulder being touched as these were close to his central venous catheter. Because he would not let the therapist work on that side of his body, his mother was instructed on using the technique, starting with the lower back and moving up until she reached the shoulder.

After a few weeks, the mother reported that she was able to begin working on the left side of his body, resulting in improved balance of his shoulders. The mother reported tremendous progress in his gait and foot strength. She observed that the reflexology and massage helped his physical body and also calmed him down before coming to the treatment centre. He looked forward to seeing the massage therapist during his weekly visits; he would immediately stick out his foot for a massage and ask to play the 'push' game.

## Movement therapies

The benefit of movement therapies among patients undergoing treatment for cancer has been documented (Bower *et al.* 2005). Yoga, karate, pilates, tai chi, or dance can all be taught to children. Movement therapies, which do not need to be rigorous in nature to provide a clinical benefit, are ideal for children undergoing extended hospital stays or those who have developed significant fatigue, reduced muscle tone, anxiety, or depression. The choice of movement therapy should take account of the child's pre-existing physical state, interests, and any complications from therapy. Movement therapies can be modified for patients who are non-ambulatory. Creating challenges, goals, or games will help capture and retain the child's interest. Repetition of movements or therapies should be cycled in order to assist with compliance. Meditation instruction may also help support lifestyle change and adherence to the movement protocols. Relaxation techniques have also been found to reduce anxiety in patients receiving chemotherapy (Deng and Cassileth 2005).

### Case 3

A 15-year-old female with ALL experienced low self-esteem, anxiety, insomnia, and body image issues during the course of her chemotherapy. To help cope with these symptoms, and especially to integrate back into the high school setting, she agreed to participate in a combined exercise and mindfulness meditation course.

The 6-week program consisted of three 2-week blocks each of (1) daily body scan meditation, (2) alternate walking and sitting meditation, and (3) gentle Hatha yoga. She was also introduced to selected mindfulness poetry. Mindfulness meditation was complemented by yoga. She was guided through a series of yoga postures while the practitioner palmed along her energy lines and pressure points, the objective being to relieve anxiety and improve overall self-esteem. A pleasant/unpleasant events calendar was completed during the first 2 weeks to monitor her progress. She reported that these therapies helped her to control her anxiety and accept the side effects associated with ALL treatment, and provided support to integrate back into high school.

## Herbal/nutrition supplements

Herbal and nutritional supplements are among the most common CAM therapies used by children with cancer. Since most patients combine the use of these supplements with conventional medicine, the healthcare provider is faced with balancing patient requests with the risk of potential adverse or beneficial interactions that may affect prognosis. The risk of CAM interacting with conventional therapy is much greater when CAM is used during the entire treatment plan. Providers should consider the desired duration of supplementation in relation to the timing of the conventional chemotherapy or radiotherapy. Careful assessment of the pharmacokinetics of the dietary supplements and the conventional chemotherapy to minimize risk of interactions may be a useful approach (Seely *et al.* 2007).

Adherence to CAM regimens that include biological agents can be challenging for children. Protocols that require restricted diets, consumption of numerous supplements, or administration through alternative routes such as inhalation or suppositories may not be feasible. Regimens that require the child to ingest multiple supplements may interfere with regular food intake and have an adverse effect on nutritional status. Development of nausea or vomiting, severe stomatitis, or cachexia should be monitored closely to ensure that the supplementary regimens are not contributing to any chemotherapy-related toxicities. Risks and benefits of the regimen as well as its effect on the child's quality of life should be discussed in detail with the family.

Caution is also advised in patients requiring nutritional intervention. Although supplements may be administered through a nasogastric tube or gastrostomy tube, the family must be educated on adequate flushing and cleaning techniques in order to avoid the risks of clogging or infection. A nutritionist should be consulted to ensure that the supplements do not interfere with the patient's planned feeding schedule or administration of conventional medications.

Data from evidence-based studies for the use of nutritional supplements in children with cancer is limited. However, studies have shown safety and potential roles for L-carnitine, glutamine, whey protein, probiotics, Traumeel S®, and essential fatty acids in children (Ladas *et al.* 2006). Herbal supplements such as echinacea, ginger, chamomile, valerian, Aloe vera, and lavender have been traditionally used in paediatrics, although research data is limited. Interest in the nutritional supplement, tolerance, risk of interactions, and prognosis should all be considered prior to the initiation of any nutritional or herbal agent.

## CAM and survivors of childhood cancer

As the conventional treatment of children with cancer becomes more effective, the challenges of survivorship have become a priority for research. Studies have estimated that 60–70% of children will have at least one disability as a result of cancer therapy; for example, they may be challenged by fatigue, pain, and anxiety and be at increased risk for heart disease, osteoporosis, infertility, and secondary malignancies (Oeffinger and Hudson 2004). Surveys on survivors of adult cancers have found that the use of CAM extends into survivorship (Boon *et al.* 2003; Hann *et al.* 2005). This trend has also been observed in survivors of childhood cancer, who report that they use CAM to reduce risk of relapse, cope with late effects from cancer therapy, or reduce their risk of developing these.

Although no research has been carried out to investigate the efficacy of CAM among survivors of childhood cancer, CAM as a component of a healthy lifestyle may provide support in coping with the late effects. Certain therapies may be of specific benefit to this population (Ladas *et al.* 2006). For example, yoga and meditation may help them cope with anxiety about cancer recurrence, and disturbances in balance or gait, or aid in maintaining a healthy weight. Acupuncture may provide relief from fatigue, pain, infertility, or disturbances in hormone balance. Some nutrition supplements may have a role in the survivor population as there is less of a concern for interactions with conventional medications.

## CAM and palliative care

Conventional therapy alone cannot always eliminate pain and suffering at the end of a child's life. Many families report that anorexia, nausea, vomiting, constipation, and diarrhoea are not adequately treated by conventional means (Wolfe *et al.* 2000). By parental report, 89% of children suffered 'a lot or a great deal' within the last month of life and the most common symptoms included fatigue, pain, dyspnoea, anorexia, nausea and vomiting, constipation, and diarrhoea. Of these symptoms, the most commonly treated were pain (76%) and dyspnoea (65%) but the response rate to conventional therapies was only 27% for pain and 16% for dyspnoea. CAM may, therefore, be useful in this setting.

Palliative care should include interventions offered to parents and siblings, as well as other caregivers, who can suffer both psychological and physical distress at the end of the child's life and subsequently in bereavement (Anghelescu *et al.* 2006). To provide optimal palliative care for children with advancing cancer, innovative interdisciplinary approaches are recommended (Beider 2005). The integration of CAM modalities into accepted practice in the care of the child suffering with unresponsive cancer provides an opportunity for each of the two traditions of healthcare to work together and learn from each other. Symptom management that utilizes integrated therapies and interventions that focus on the child as a whole human being and not just one symptom at a time is highly recommended (Anghelescù *et al.* 2006).

## Conclusion

The use of CAM among children with cancer is increasing, especially in cases where conventional therapies have proved ineffective in controlling symptoms or preventing progression of the disease. Despite greater interest among conventional practitioners in researching this field, there is insufficient evidence to guide discussions on many of these therapies, especially the biological ones. However, some types such as acupuncture, massage, and movement therapies are known to be beneficial for managing complications of conventional treatment. The International Society of Pediatric Oncology has developed guidelines to enhance communication between healthcare providers and families on the use of these therapies. The guidelines call for the healthcare team to be attentive to CAM therapies that may be physically or psychologically harmful to children and their families but not to automatically and dismissively discourage the use of non-harmful ones (Jankovic *et al.* 2004).

## References

Ahles, T. A., Tope, D. M., Pinkson, B. *et al.* 1999, Massage therapy for patients undergoing autologous bone marrow transplantation, *Journal of Pain and Symptom Management*, vol. **18**, pp. 157–63.

Anghelescu, D. L., Oakes, L. & Hinds, P. S. 2006, Palliative care and pediatrics, *Anesthesiology Clinics of North America*, vol. **24**, pp. 145–61.

Beachy, J. M. 2003, Premature infant massage in the NICU, *Neonatal Network*, vol. **22**, pp. 39–45.

Beider, S. 2005, An ethical argument for integrated palliative care, *Evidence-Based Complementary and Alternative Medicine*, vol. **2**, pp. 27–31.

Boon, H., Westlake, K., Stewart, M. *et al.* 2003, Use of complementary/alternative medicine by men diagnosed with prostate cancer: prevalence and characteristics, *Urology*, vol. **62**, pp. 849–53.

Bower, J. E., Woolery, A., Sternlieb, B. & Garet, D. 2005, Yoga for cancer patients and survivors, *Cancer Control*, vol. **12**, pp. 165–71.

Deng, G. & Cassileth, B. R. 2005, Integrative oncology: complementary therapies for pain, anxiety, and mood disturbance, *CA: A Cancer Journal for Clinicians*, vol. **55**, pp. 109–16.

Hann, D., Baker, F., Denniston, M. & Entrekin, N. 2005, Long-term breast cancer survivors' use of complementary therapies: perceived impact on recovery and prevention of recurrence, *Integrative Cancer Therapies*, vol. **4**, pp. 14–20.

Jankovic, M., Spinetta, J.J., Martins, A.G. *et al.* 2004, Non-conventional therapies in childhood cancer: Guidelines for distinguishing non-harmful from harmful therapies: A report of the SIOP working committee on psychological issues in pediatric oncology, *Pediatric Blood and Cancer*, vol. **42**, pp. 106–8.

Johnstone, P. A., Niemtzow, R. C. & Riffenburgh, R. H. 2002, Acupuncture for xerostomia: clinical update, *Cancer*, vol. **94**, pp. 1151–56.

Kelly, K. M. 2004, Complementary and alternative medical therapies for children with cancer, *European Journal of Cancer*, vol. **40**, pp. 2041–46.

Kemper, K. J., Sarah, R., Silver-Highfield, E., Xiarhos, E., Barnes, L. & Berde, C. 2000, On pins and needles? Pediatric pain patients' experience with acupuncture, *Pediatrics*, vol. **105**, pp. 941–47.

Ladas, E. J., Post-White, J., Hawkes, R. & Taromina, K. 2006, Evidence for symptom management in the child with cancer, *Journal of Pediatric Hematology/Oncology*, vol. **28**, pp. 601–15.

Loman, D. 2006, The use of complementary and alternative health care practices among children, *Journal of Pediatric Health Care*, vol. **17**, pp. 58–63.

Oeffinger, K. C. & Hudson, M. M. 2004, Long-term complications following childhood and adolescent cancer: foundations for providing risk-based health care for survivors, *CA: A Cancer Journal for Clinicians*, vol. **54**, pp. 208–36.

Reindl, T. K., Geilen, W., Hartmann, R. *et al.* 2006, Acupuncture against chemotherapy-induced nausea and vomiting in pediatric oncology. Interim results of a multicenter crossover study, *Supportive Care in Cancer*, vol. **14**, pp. 172–76.

Seely, D., Stempak, D. & Baruchel, S. 2007, A strategy for controlling potential interactions between natural health products and chemotherapy: A review in pediatric oncology, *Journal of Pediatric Hematology/Oncology*, vol. **29**, pp. 32–47.

Taromina, K., Ladas, E. J., Rooney, D., Hughes, D. & Kelly, K. M. 2006, A retrospective review investigating the feasibility of acupuncture as a supportive care agent in a pediatric oncology service. Society for Integrative Oncology, Annual Meeting, November 9, 2006.

Vickers, A. J., Straus, D. J., Fearon, B. & Cassileth, B. R. 2004, Acupuncture for postchemotherapy fatigue: a phase II study, *Journal of Clinical Oncology*, vol. **22**, pp. 1731–35.

Wolfe, J., Grier, H. E., Klar, N. *et al.* 2000, Symptoms and suffering at the end of life in children with cancer, *New England Journal of Medicine*, vol. **342**, pp. 326–33.

Chapter 7

# Choice and co-ordination of therapies: the family doctor as guide

Catherine Zollman

## Summary

The task of navigating the maze of potential CAM treatments and integrating CAM into a personal cancer care plan is often complex, time-consuming, and stressful. It can also be empowering, health enhancing, and life transforming. A trusted and wise guide can provide valuable support for people along this journey. There are many facets to the role of a guide, depending on the individuals concerned and their circumstances. These might include helping them decide what they want from CAM, finding the right therapy and therapist, evaluating CAM interventions, preventing adverse effects, and co-ordinating their care while keeping sight of the bigger picture. Family doctors have a range of skills and attributes that make them eminently suited to being such a guide and this can be a tremendously satisfying and rewarding role.

## Introduction

People often say that the diagnosis of cancer launches them onto a conveyor belt, carrying them along on a journey where they feel they have very little control or choice. The decision to incorporate one or more complementary approaches into a cancer journey can be a reaction to this, a deliberate step to regain some control and make some choices. However, having choices comes hand-in-hand with a need to make decisions and decisions about complementary cancer treatments are not always easy or straightforward. They may have major lifestyle or financial implications, or risk straying into unknown, unresearched, and potentially health-compromising territories. Where can people turn for help?

There is no shortage of information; a basic Internet search of complementary medicine in cancer brings up more than 8.5 million hits. So, where to start? Since conventional sources of cancer care information (consultants, medical journals, research databases, etc.) have not traditionally included advice about CAM, people usually have to 'go it alone' in trying to sift helpful from unhelpful information. For the person, or a closely involved supporter, coming to terms with a diagnosis of cancer, this can seem a lonely and unsupported task, a huge responsibility, and another significant source of stress. In this situation, wise and impartial guidance from a trusted source can have a major positive impact. Such guidance might help individuals weigh up options, think through the likely impact of various choices, pace, evaluate, and co-ordinate various activities, and consider a wider perspective. Having a 'bad' guide is probably worse than having no guide at all, and therefore it becomes all the more important to find a 'good' one.

## Key characteristics of a guide

I have drawn the following list from surveys of the support and information needs of patients with cancer (Mackenzie *et al.* 1999; Verhoef *et al.* 1999; Sleath *et al.* 2005) and from conversations with people with cancer and their supporters over the last 16 years. Considering the key characteristics of a good guide, firstly and most importantly there must be trust. This could have been built up over years or could be the result of a good first meeting where a person feels he/she has been truly heard and understood and where the guide's responses seem congruent with, or at least supportive of, his/her own views. A guide must also be able to stand back from his or her own agenda and 'get alongside' the person with cancer, really seeing things from that person's perspective. This requires both impartiality and empathy. Therefore, ideally, a guide should not be directly involved in providing any particular aspect of cancer care but should have some understanding of all the different providers involved. He or she should be non-judgmental and accepting of wherever the persons with cancer find themselves in terms of emotional, physical, mental, and spiritual orientation. It is also important that a guide be comfortable dealing with uncertainty, experienced at helping people assess the risks and benefits of various treatment options, and flexible in approach. He/she must be honest but with an ability to maintain an appropriate sense of hope (Verhoef *et al.* 1999). Extensive knowledge of CAM is not expected or essential. More important is that the guide should demonstrate a real interest in the individual as a person, not just as a patient with cancer. Good communication skills and a participatory decision-making style are also highly valued (Sleath *et al.* 2005). Of fundamental importance is the ability of a guide to support without taking control and without undermining the person's autonomy to decide his or her own path.

## Family doctors as guides

### Why might a family doctor make a good guide?

Interestingly, all the features of a guide listed earlier are also many of the key skills and attributes that characterize a good family doctor. In the UK, the General Practice curriculum and the General Medical Council's guidance for doctors (General Medical Council 2001; Royal College of General Practitioners 2006) emphasize trustworthiness, empathy, respect, and impartiality as core elements. Family doctor training programmes in other countries too usually include communication skills and patient-centred consulting. The fact that a family doctor is available, accessible, and local and often has a pre-existing relationship with the person, which includes an understanding of their family and social backgrounds, is also a potential asset (Brennan *et al.* 2006). In many aspects of conventional healthcare, the family doctor's role is one of a co-ordinator and a trusted adviser and this should theoretically be extendable to incorporate the role of CAM cancer care guide. So, one place to seek a guide is in one's local family doctor or possibly in another member of the primary health care team. That being said, there are also a number of factors that may make it difficult for family doctors to fulfil this role or for persons with cancer to feel that their family doctor is the most appropriate guide for them.

### Barriers to family doctors becoming guides

Time constraints are a major factor in influencing people's decisions to open up and form a trusting relationship and in influencing any doctor's decision about whether or not to take on a guiding or advocacy role. Being clear about exactly what is expected and what is available can be very helpful and can enable family doctors to play a useful role without feeling a risk of unsustainable demand or dependence. Some primary care doctors feel ambivalent, indifferent, or even opposed to CAM. Although people are not necessarily seeking expert knowledge of CAM, some family doctors consider themselves too ill informed to enter into discussions about their patients' hopes and concerns on this subject. Many family doctors feel most comfortable taking an evidence-based approach and as the evidence base for CAM in cancer treatment is still in its infancy, they feel unable to offer support in this field (Tasaki *et al.* 2002). Also, once care is taken over by hospital specialists, family doctors can sometimes find themselves marginalized and out of touch with a person's individual cancer journey, especially if a large number of other healthcare workers are involved (Norman *et al.* 2001). It may require a proactive approach to keep in touch and maintain good lines of communication with all parties involved. People prefer their family doctors to be advocates rather than gatekeepers (Bain *et al.* 2002), so one who is perceived as a potential barrier to obtaining access to specialist treatment may not do well in a guiding role. If there was any problem or delay with the initial diagnosis of cancer, damage may already have been done to the doctor–patient relationship. In some instances, this can lead to a permanent breakdown of trust, even extending to other doctors or staff in the same practice. However, if the barriers listed earlier can be overcome, there is a real opportunity for a motivated family doctor to make a unique and valuable contribution, which can spread beyond the individual person with cancer and benefit the person's family and others involved in his/her cancer journey.

## Roles of a guide

### Helping people work out what they want

So, what is involved in being a guide for someone who wishes to integrate CAM into his or her cancer care? First and foremost, it is about helping that person decide their aims. It is easy to assume that anyone looking to CAM is harbouring unrealistic hopes of cure, but in practice there are many other reasons (Correa-Velez *et al.* 2005). Some might be seeking symptom control, either for the cancer itself or for side effects of treatment. Others might want to address their human or existential concerns. Help with relaxation and stress management for themselves and others is another reason, as is wanting to maximize the body's self-healing and immune responses. Some people are looking for a transformational experience—wanting to re-evaluate and re-orientate their lives in the light of their cancer diagnosis. In addition, there can be other more individual reasons as well. Sometimes people with cancer have already become very clear about their reasons, either rationally or through a more intuitive process. In other cases, there may be only an ill-defined sense of what they want. Some people might need a guide's support to reject CAM if they are being pressurized to use it by friends or family. However, when they are coming to their decisions, a guide can take the role of active and reflective listener to help them clarify, reality-check, and confirm their goals.

### Weighing up options

Once clear about where they are aiming for, people with cancer often find themselves faced with a large number of possible routes to get there. A phase of information gathering is usually necessary, followed by a period of weighing up the various options. A guide may be able to recommend some trustworthy sources of information but often the problem is not a lack but an overwhelming excess of information. Therefore, a more useful role is to help clarify, again using reflective listening skills and exploratory questioning, as to which of the various options available is most likely to fulfil the unique needs of the individual concerned. This process may involve helping someone think through the likely short-, medium-, and even long-term impacts of various choices, both on themselves and on their close supporters. If there is a major discrepancy in the weighting of different options by the person with cancer and his or her supporters or if the guide feels strongly that someone is making a decision that will compromise his or her health (and health in this context is meant in its broadest sense incorporating social, physical, mental, and spiritual aspects), this presents an enormous challenge. Although respecting patient autonomy is an ethical and medico-legal duty of any doctor and a fundamental role of a cancer guide, research shows that in practice there is a shift in many (especially hospital-based) doctors' respect for an individual's autonomy in refusing treatment options that are considered curative (van Kleffens *et al.* 2004). The amount of pressure that a physician will exert to influence whether or not someone will agree to undergo curative treatment will vary depending on individual circumstances but it is helpful for all parties to be aware of this 'respect shift' and perhaps discuss it openly during the options appraisal phase. For a guide, this will undoubtedly require trust, honesty, and mutual respect if the relationship is to be maintained.

## Finding the right therapy

It might be assumed that, once someone has decided what they would like to achieve through using CAM, it should be simple to decide which therapy would be most suitable. Unfortunately, it is not that easy! Because there is no one-to-one matching of clinical condition or symptom with most appropriate therapy and there is often a broad overlap between the claims of different CAM disciplines, it becomes more a matter of individual choice. Many factors will influence that choice: whether someone prefers taking a 'medicine' by mouth (e.g. homeopathy, herbal medicine, nutritional medicine), receiving physical treatments (e.g. massage, shiatsu, osteopathy, cransiosacral therapy, acupuncture), actively engaging the mind–body connection (e.g. hypnosis, autogenic training, biofeedback, relaxation), or physical exercise including breathing techniques (e.g. yoga, tai chi, qi gong, Alexander Technique, Feldenkrais).

Personal experience of a therapy or anecdotal experience of friends or relatives will also influence a person's decisions, although the flip side of this is that a person with cancer may feel pressured to make choices that are more about others' interests than his or her own. A guide can help people see this anecdotal information in a broader context alongside other types of information.

Sometimes there is research evidence that helps one to guide decisions, but for many clinical scenarios, there is no specific evidence on CAM or the evidence base reflects those therapies that are easiest to research rather than those that are most effective.

Sometimes, the person's physical or emotional state dictates which type of therapy will be most suitable. If someone has low energy during or following chemo- or radiotherapy, it may be inappropriate to advise a challenging physical exercise regimen, major dietary shift, or mind–body therapy requiring focused concentration. The presence of pain and the need for analgesia can also influence what is possible. Depression (a common associated diagnosis in people with cancer) may reduce levels of motivation and so rule out certain self-help approaches. In other words, a guide may have a role in helping people with cancer match their choice of CAM therapy with their state of health.

Access to and funding for CAM are other factors that will have a major influence on a person's choice. A local therapist who is experienced in dealing with people with cancer and who has good links with the conventional oncology services might be an appropriate choice, whichever therapy he/she may practice. If there is NHS provision of a CAM therapy or a subsidized or free local service, it may be appropriate to choose this initially rather than increasing financial stresses. Flexibility of access to a therapy, such as where and when it is available, is another consideration. Often, people feel that they have to have 'the best' therapy and will often go to great lengths and compromise other aspects of their life and health to achieve this. A guide's reassurance that 'best' is a multi-faceted description, and that a local therapy that does not make them exhausted may actually be better than a famous one that is more difficult to access, may give relief and remove an unnecessary heavy burden of duty.

## Finding the right therapist

Notwithstanding issues of access and funding, it does appear important to most CAM users that the therapist they consult is someone they can trust and respect. A guide can help clarify expectations in this regard, encourage people to trust their instincts and reactions in trying out various therapists and in deciding whether or not to opt for ongoing treatment and help them to be 'street-wise' about their use of CAM. This often requires specific encouragement as there is sometimes a belief that it is necessary to suspend critical faculties before entering into a CAM therapeutic relationship—for example, not questioning the recommended duration or frequency of treatments or the explanations of illness causation put forward. Hopefully, an open, interactive relationship will evolve between the client and therapist, where the experience and the expertise of both the parties are valued and both feel part of a therapeutic partnership. A guide may be able to spot where a relationship with a practitioner is becoming unhelpful, for example, by colluding in denial or by fostering dependence, and reflect this back to the user.

## Helping to evaluate CAM interventions

It is impossible to predict the result of any given CAM intervention in an individual case. Even if a therapy is beneficial in some way, if it is difficult to tolerate or is difficult to access or maintain, it may not be in the individual's best interests to continue. For example, although a Chinese herbal decoction may be helpful, the taste or smell may be too unpleasant. Sometimes the sheer number of tablets they are already taking puts people off oral nutritional or other supplements. The cost and time commitment of pursuing a particular CAM therapy must also be weighed against the subjective and objective benefits observed. Often, a few trial sessions will give someone a sense of whether a therapy will be helpful in their current situation but sometimes the close relationship between the client and the CAM practitioner makes it difficult to stand back and evaluate the therapy critically—is it really doing me any good? Answering this is often made harder by the fact that many CAM therapies aim to give results in the longer term, promoting wellness as opposed to taking away particular symptoms. It can be difficult to decide whether to continue a therapy if there are no immediate effects to assess, only the possibility of some health gain in the future. A good guide can therefore help a person to develop realistic time frames and some clearly thought-through markers with which to decide how beneficial a particular therapy is for him/her. A guide who is outside the immediate situation can often observe more clearly the full effects of a therapy, whereas a patient or their supporters may have their objectivity clouded by their fervent desire for a positive outcome. If there is a difference in the perception of benefit between client, supporter, and guide, this will need very careful and sensitive handling and ultimately respect for an individual's autonomous decisions once they have been adequately informed.

## Monitoring for adverse effects of CAM—specific and non-specific

People tend to think of CAM therapies as safe and where they are used appropriately, this is usually the case. However, something with the potential to do good may also do harm so it is a useful role of any guide to raise awareness of the risks and help monitor any treatment for potential adverse effects. Risks can be considered under two headings—specific adverse effects of individual therapies and non-specific adverse effects of CAM in general.

### Specific adverse effects

Each therapy will have its own potential complications and contra-indications. For example, acupuncture can cause local bleeding, bruising, and temporary light-headedness. In very rare instances, and usually in inexperienced hands, serious adverse events such as needling of the chest wall causing pneumothorax have been reported. Experienced practitioners will warn clients about potential adverse effects and follow guidelines as to the suitability of their treatments in individual circumstances. The general common-sense advice is to avoid situations that might aggravate an underlying condition, for example, avoiding strong manipulation or massage directly over the site of any active cancer lesion, deep venous thrombosis, or radiotherapy-sensitized skin. Manipulation of people with any form of bone cancer should be avoided because of the risk of fractures. Direct toxic effects from herbal medicines are possible; contaminated or inappropriate herbs have caused serious, sometimes fatal, organ damage. Herbal remedies and some nutritional supplements can interact pharmacologically with conventional medication and have damaging results. People undergoing treatment for cancer are often prescribed complex regimens of multiple medicines. Predicting the potential interactions with herbal medicine requires great expertise and so a guide should encourage such people not to self-medicate and only to take additional medicines or supplements on the advice of a registered practitioner who is very experienced in the field of cancer and who has access to the various databases of drug–herb interactions. Monitoring biochemical markers, such as liver or kidney function tests, can be helpful.

## Non-specific adverse effects

Using CAM can have a range of other negative consequences that have nothing to do with the specific therapy being used but result from the act of choosing and using CAM in general. Some of these are logical consequences of the very aspects of CAM that make it attractive to many users.

◆ *Empowerment versus guilt and burden of responsibility*: Choosing CAM can often give people a sense of empowerment and increased control as they take more responsibility for the management of their illness, rather than passively accepting what their doctors recommend. The negative corollary of this is that if the clinical condition deteriorates, there can be a burden of guilt and a feeling of being personally responsible for the deterioration—'*If only I had meditated more…*' or '*If only I had stopped drinking coffee…*'. Even more pernicious is the fact that some people come away with the belief that it is their personality or their life choices that are responsible for their cancer. Once this idea is ingrained, they can find it hard to stop focusing on a past that might have been different and to start living in the present in the best and most health-giving way possible.

◆ *Missed diagnosis or 'masked' symptoms*: Another non-specific effect that often concerns doctors is the possibility that CAM treatments might alleviate symptoms and mask an important diagnosis, such as intercurrent infection or imminent cord compression, which requires urgent conventional treatment. Guides should encourage all people pursuing an integrated or complementary approach to maintain contact with, and report changing symptoms to, both the conventional and CAM practitioners involved in their care.

◆ *Problems associated with stopping conventional medication*: Sometimes people using CAM decide not to accept or continue with conventional anti-cancer treatments. This can be for a variety of reasons: a philosophical rejection of the idea of introducing toxic chemicals or radiation into the body, a previous bad experience of conventional medicine, personal experience of side effects, or a realistic appraisal that the risks of the treatments offered outweigh the likely benefits. Sometimes a CAM practitioner tells, or is believed to have told, someone to stop conventional medication. Whatever the reasons behind the refusal of potentially beneficial conventional treatments, it often causes a wide range of responses and potential for major conflict in all those involved, from doctors and nurses to family members. If a family doctor guide feels that stopping beneficial medication could present a genuine health risk, they should encourage exploration and supportively challenge the reasons behind the decision and ensure and document that the person is adequately informed. Where it is possible to have an open discussion considering the perspectives of all concerned, the reasons behind any decisions, and the person's expectations of the chosen treatment methods, this can reduce the tension. A guide can help by encouraging such a discussion and possibly by preparing the ground with some of the interested parties, acting as an advocate or supporter.

## Co-ordinating care—seeing the big picture, maintaining ongoing contact

As today's cancer care is such a specialized field with surgeons, clinical oncologists, and medical oncologists all taking centre stage at one point or another and these episodes often being interspersed with long periods of 'watchful waiting' with much less frequent hospital visits, it is not uncommon for the person with cancer and their close supporters to feel that they are the only ones with a clear picture of the cancer journey as a whole. This can be lonely and frustrating. It can also feel disorientating as the characters, who for intense periods of time become all-powerful central figures, seem to withdraw from reach once a particular treatment is complete. There can be feelings of abandonment and rejection or even of grieving for the loss of a relationship with an individual trusted professional. A guide who is there through the various episodes along the journey, whose perspective encompasses the bigger picture, and whose involvement is not dependent on any particular phase of treatment or follow-up can provide the continuity necessary to ensure smoothly co-ordinated and individually tailored care. In particular, he or she will be able to help people decide about their ongoing use of CAM, reduce the chances of fragmentation of care, and monitor any signs of CAM use leading to or exacerbating denial.

## Ongoing CAM treatment: potential dependence and financial implications

When a treatment is considered health promoting rather than symptom or disease relieving, it is difficult to know how much is sufficient. Many practitioners advocate 'top-up' treatments for patients once an initial course is complete. Given that there is always room for improvement in health, that many CAM treatments cause a beneficial placebo and relaxation response, and that having regular CAM can be seen as a kind of (unproven) insurance policy against future problems, it is difficult to draw the line between an appropriate and useful amount of health-maintenance behaviour and an unhelpful pattern of dependence or even financial exploitation. A guide has a valuable role in helping people evaluate the ongoing role of CAM in their lives, including the financial implications, and in helping them distinguish between the positive and negative reasons for continuing.

## Discouraging fragmentation of care

CAM happens largely outside the NHS; therefore, information may not be communicated to conventional healthcare workers unless it is via the people with cancer themselves. This is a missed opportunity for sharing useful information—for example, CAM practitioners often enquire in depth and therefore have a detailed understanding of a person's background and personality, which could help conventional healthcare workers in many ways, for example, with concordance and other psychosocial aspects of care. Where care is fragmented and interprofessional communication is poor, unhelpful situations involving, for example, contradictory information or potentially hazardous treatment interactions become more likely. Family doctors recognize this (O'Beirne *et al.* 2004) and can encourage information sharing directly between the professionals involved or can at least act as a professional intermediary to oversee, if not help coordinate, the total package of care.

## Giving hope versus generating false hope and encouraging denial

Even if this is not their main or only reason, many people who seek CAM as a part of a package of cancer care are hoping to improve their prognosis

(Correa-Velez *et al.* 2005). Given that having a sense of hope increases quality of life and conversely that feelings of hopelessness reduce quality of life, this can be seen as a positive step. On the other hand, it can be part of an unhealthy pattern of denial, a disconnection from reality, and an avoidance of some of the necessary stages of adjustment and acceptance that can help people really 'live well' with cancer. Penny Brohn, the founder of the Bristol Cancer Help Centre who died from metastatic breast cancer after several relapses, said towards the end of her life, 'I still believe there is no such thing as false hope'— meaning, I believe, that one can always hope for something and that being able to find a path to hope, which does not necessarily mean denying the facts of one's illness, can be a life-enhancing and sustaining process. A guide who can help people navigate and balance through this difficult and narrow terrain is playing a very valuable role indeed.

## References

Bain, N. S. C., Campbell, N. C., Ritchie, L. D. & Cassidy, J. 2002, Striking the right balance in colorectal cancer care – a qualitative study of rural and urban patients, *Family Practice*, vol. **19**, no. 4, pp. 369–74.

Brennan, M., Black, E., French, J. & Boyages, J. 2006, Breast cancer - guiding your patient through treatment, *Australian Family Physician*, vol. **35**, no. 3, pp. 117–20.

Correa-Velez, I., Clavarino, A. & Eastwood, H. 2005, Surviving, relieving, repairing, and boosting up: reasons for using complementary/alternative medicine among patients with advanced cancer: a thematic analysis, *Journal of Palliative Medicine*, vol. **8**, no. 5, pp. 953–61.

General Medical Council 2001, *Good Medical Practice* 3rd edn, GMC, London.

Mackenzie, G., Parkinson, M., Lakhani, A. & Pannekoek, H. 1999, Issues that influence patient/physician discussion of complementary therapies, *Patient Education and Counselling*, vol. **38**, no. 2, pp. 155–9.

Norman, A., Sisler, J., Hack, T. & Harlos, M. 2001, Family physicians and cancer care. Palliative care patients' perspectives, *Canadian Family Physician*, vol. **47**, pp. 2009–12, 2015–6.

O'Beirne, M., Verhoef, M., Paluck, E. & Herbert, C. 2004, Complementary therapy use by cancer patients. Physician' perceptions, attitudes and ideas, *Canadian Family Physician*, vol. **50**, pp. 882–8.

Royal College of General Practitioners. 2006, Curriculum Statement 1: Being a General Practitioner. RCGP, 4 Princes Gate, Hyde Park, London.

Sleath, B., Callahan, L., DeVellis, R. F., Sloane, P. D. 2005, Patients' perceptions of primary care physicans' participatory decision-making style and communication about complementary and alternative medicine for arthritis, *Journal of Alternative and Complementary Medicine*, vol. **11**, no. 3, pp. 449–53.

Tasaki, K., Maskarinec, G., Shumay, D. M., Tatsumura, Y. & Kakai, H. 2002, Communication between physicians and cancer patients about complementary and alternative medicine: exploring patients' perspectives, *Psycho-oncology*, vol. **11**, no. 3, pp. 212–20.

van Kleffens, T., van Baarsen, B. & van Leeuwen, E. 2004, The medical practice of patient autonomy and cancer treatment refusals: a patients' and physicians' perspective, *Social Science and Medicine*, vol. **58**, no. 11, pp. 2325–36.

Verhoef, M. J., White, M. A. & Doll, R. 1999, Cancer patients' expectations of the role of family physicians in communication about complementary therapies, *Cancer Prevention and Control*, vol. **3**, no. 3, pp. 181–7.

Chapter 8

# Acupuncture

Beverley de Valois

## Summary

Acupuncture is a therapeutic technique that evolved from ancient Oriental theories and practices of medicine. Since the 1970s, it has become increasingly popular in the West as a means of preventing and treating a variety of disorders. In cancer care, it is used to complement conventional management, helping to control cancer symptoms and the side effects of treatment, as well as being used in the supportive care of people with cancer. It is suitable at any stage of the cancer experience, from diagnosis through active treatment, in palliative and end of life care, and to support survivors in re-establishing their lives.

## Definition

Acupuncture may be defined as a family of procedures used to stimulate specific sites on the body known as acupuncture points. Needling is the most common and well-known means of stimulation used in acupuncture and involves the insertion of thin, solid metallic needles under the surface of the skin. These needles are sometimes stimulated manually or with electrical currents (electroacupuncture). Other techniques used to stimulate acupuncture points include heat (including moxibustion, the burning of the herb *Artemesia vulgaris*, commonly known as mugwort), cupping, laser, and acupressure, as well as interventions such as transcutaneous electrical nerve stimulation (TENS) and devices such as sea bands. This chapter focuses primarily on the use of needling and moxibustion, as used in traditional forms of acupuncture.

## History

Acupuncture is part of traditional Chinese medicine, whose medical theories have been under continuous development for more than 3000 years. Acupuncture itself may have emerged during 200–100 BCE (Birch and Felt 1999). Evolving over many centuries, its practice spread to neighbouring countries including Japan, Korea, Vietnam, and Taiwan, where it was adapted to suit local conditions. It first appeared in the West as early as the mid-seventeenth century but it was not until President Nixon's visit to China in 1972 that it caught the interest of Western healthcare practitioners. Today, acupuncture is practised and is gaining acceptance worldwide. The World Health Organisation (2003) recognized the 'promising potential' of acupuncture for relieving pain and nausea and the National Institutes of Health (NIH) (1997) concluded that there were promising results for the efficacy of acupuncture in postoperative and chemotherapy nausea and vomiting, as well as indications for its use in a range of other conditions. In the United Kingdom, the House of Lords Select Committee on Science and Technology (2000) included acupuncture as one of the 'Big Five' principle disciplines in their classification of complementary and alternative medicines.

Acupuncture practice has adapted as it crossed national boundaries, making it a richly diverse practice. In the West, acupuncture can be broadly classified into two distinct styles: traditional acupuncture and Western medical acupuncture.

## Modes of action

### Traditional acupuncture

Traditional acupuncture has evolved over the centuries from the theories of Chinese medicine. These are based on the concept that *qi* (pronounced chee), or energy, flows through the body. A simplified explanation of the relation of *qi* to health is that when *qi* flows through the body smoothly, then wellness is maintained. However, if the flow of *qi* is disturbed, then symptoms result. Factors that can affect the flow of *qi* include emotional states (such as anger, fear, and worry), poor nutrition, overwork, trauma, or exposure to climactic factors such as cold or damp. Stimulating energy in the acupuncture points influences the behaviour of the *qi*, with the aim of restoring its normal flow to rebalance the body to reduce or eliminate manifestations of ill health.

The complex theories of traditional Chinese medicine require detailed understanding of the functions of the organs, the 14 ordinary and 8 extraordinary channels (or pathways) through which the *qi* flows and the acupuncture points themselves (of which there are about 500). Fundamental to the idea of *qi* are the concepts of *yin* and *yang*, two qualities that reflect the opposing, dynamic, and transforming nature of *qi* and the five phases or elements. These concepts underpin the notion of *qi* as a dynamic that moves or flows according to specific patterns or cycles. Through understanding the nature of *qi*, its patterns, and influences, traditional acupuncturists work to identify an individual's specific imbalances. They devise appropriate treatment plans that use selected acupuncture points to improve the flow of *qi* and restore or improve well-being.

Because of the complex web formed by the relationships of the organs and channels, the acupuncture points selected to treat a particular condition may be located some distance from the area where the complaint manifests. For instance, some types of headaches are treated primarily using points on the feet or arms. Similarly, conditions of the breast may be treated using acupuncture points on the feet, arms, or the upper back (it is contraindicated to needle into breast tissue).

There are various styles of traditional acupuncture, each of which has its own characteristics. Examples include Japanese acupuncture, Korean acupuncture, Traditional Chinese Medicine (TCM), Eight Principles acupuncture, and five elements acupuncture.

## Western medical acupuncture

Western medical acupuncture is based on a different theoretical framework, developed over the last 30 years to suit the theories of modern conventional medicine. However, within this framework, it is still difficult to ascertain how acupuncture works. Many theories exist: some propose that it regulates the nervous system, stimulating the production of biochemicals such as endorphins and serotonin, thereby influencing perception of pain; others suggest that it affects the release of neurotransmitters and neurohormones, thus affecting the central nervous system (National Center for Complementary and Alternative Medicine 2004).

## Ear acupuncture

Ear acupuncture or auriculotherapy combines traditional and modern theoretical frameworks. In this style, it is believed that areas of the ear correspond to areas of the body and stimulation of acupuncture points on the surface of the ear can influence symptoms in the corresponding part.

## Indications

Acupuncture may be beneficial at any stage of a person's cancer experience. It can be used after diagnosis to manage shock and complex emotional reactions. It is useful for managing the symptoms of cancer and the side effects of cancer treatments, including surgery, radiotherapy, chemotherapy, and hormonal treatments. It is actively used throughout the world in palliative care and in the United Kingdom is included in the *National Guidelines for the Use of Complementary Therapies in Supportive and Palliative Care* (Tavares 2003). It may also be helpful in end-of-life treatment (Pan *et al.* 2000). Acupuncture can help survivors to adjust following cancer treatment and to re-establish a normal life. Although most research focuses on the management of physical symptoms, acupuncture can also be beneficial in helping patients cope with the strong emotions associated with their illness.

## Evidence base

Although numerous studies about using acupuncture to manage cancer-related symptoms have been published, the evidence for most applications remains inconclusive. Trial methodology for acupuncture studies is complex and many studies are deemed to have flawed methodology. Bearing this in mind, it is informative to look at the areas that have attracted research interest. In most of these cases, although results may be inconclusive, initial indications of acupuncture's effectiveness are promising and further research is warranted.

### Cancer pain

Acupuncture, particularly Western medical acupuncture, is widely used in pain clinics. In fact, the Chinese demonstrations of acupuncture used in place of anaesthesia in the 1970s are what attracted Western medical interest to acupuncture. Although acupuncture is not used for anaesthesia in the West, studies indicate that it can reduce postoperative pain, with a resulting reduction in the need for postoperative analgesics. Women undergoing axillary dissection for breast cancer experienced less pain and increased mobility when treated with acupuncture following surgery (Tavares 2003; National Cancer Institute 2005).

Research into the effectiveness of acupuncture in managing chronic and treatment-related pain is confined to observational studies, case series, and audits. There are indications that acupuncture can be useful in managing chronic pain, with resultant improvements in mobility, depression scores, and reductions in distress. However, pain control appears to become more difficult with advanced disease and tolerance to treatment may be an indicator for tumour recurrence (Tavares 2003).

### Chemotherapy-induced nausea and vomiting

Commentators agree that the evidence for the positive effects of acupuncture on chemotherapy-induced nausea and vomiting is convincing, with numerous studies providing comparable results. A systematic review (Vickers 1996, cited in Tavares 2003) concluded that although the studies examined had some methodological flaws, a particular acupuncture point—Pericardium 6 (PC6)—seems to be an effective antiemetic point. Prevention appears to be more successful than control once emesis begins and results may be short term.

## Breathlessness (dyspnoea)

Although there are relatively few trials examining the effectiveness of acupuncture to manage breathlessness, a review (Ernst 2001, cited in Tavares 2003) concluded that there was adequate data to support the use of acupuncture to relieve this symptom in end-of-life care. Two randomized controlled trials (RCTs) using traditional acupuncture and acupressure, respectively, showed that patients with chronic obstructive pulmonary disease had significant benefit over comparative groups receiving sham treatment (techniques that are not intended to stimulate known acupuncture points) (National Institutes of Health 1997). A pilot study of 20 patients with cancer-related breathlessness reported marked symptomatic improvements in 70% of the participants (Tavares 2003).

## Dry mouth (xerostomia)

Several studies indicate promising results in increasing salivary flow in patients suffering from xerostomia due to a variety of causes. Acupuncture is also helpful for patients experiencing this in late-stage palliative care (Tavares 2003).

## Hot flushes and night sweats

Several studies have investigated the use of acupuncture to manage hot flushes and night sweats in women with breast cancer and in men undergoing treatment for prostate cancer, with promising results (Smith *et al.* 2005). The author's research indicated that women taking tamoxifen experienced reductions in hot flush frequency, as well as improvements in physical and emotional well-being, after a course of acupuncture (de Valois 2006b). Many of the participants expressed a preference for managing these treatment side effects with acupuncture, rather than additional medication.

## Anxiety and depression

The hot flush study cited above showed that participants had significant reductions in levels of anxiety/fears and depressed mood measured on the Women's Health Questionnaire. Ernst *et al.* (1998) found acupuncture to be as effective as tricyclic drugs, and Gould and MacPherson (2001) noted that it is a common phenomenon for patients receiving acupuncture treatment for other conditions to report improvements in mood (cited in Tavares 2003).

## Immune function

Research in China into the effect of acupuncture on the immune system also shows promising results, with three RCTs showing enhanced immune system function and one RCT showing enhanced leukocyte phagocytic activity. These RCTs received high scores for levels of evidence when evaluated by the National Cancer Institute (2005). A further case series of 28 patients with cancer undergoing chemotherapy showed no declines in T cells and in natural killer cell activity, both of which are usually suppressed by chemotherapy (National Cancer Institute 2005).

## Other symptoms

There are published case series reports that describe clinical observations of improvements for a number of other cancer-related symptoms including rectitis, dysphonia, oesophageal obstruction, and postoperative lymphoedema (National Cancer Institute 2005), as well as radionecrotic ulcers, intractable hiccup, and uraemic pruritis (Tavares 2003).

## Treating overall well-being

While research tends to focus on acupuncture's effects on specific symptoms, acupuncture treatment has a wider effect than simply addressing the main complaint(s). It is common for patients receiving acupuncture treatment to experience improvements in a wide range of symptoms that may seem unrelated to the main ones. Participants in two observational hot flush studies recorded improvements in quality of sleep, memory and concentration, energy levels, and reduced levels of anxiety/fears, depressed mood, and somatic symptoms, in addition to reductions in hot flush frequency (de Valois 2006b).

Acupuncture may also play an important role in enhancing psychospiritual well-being (Tavares 2003). Certain forms of traditional acupuncture, such as five elements, feature treatment at emotional and spiritual levels (Hicks *et al.* 2004). Many patients find this a valuable aspect, which can be an essential feature of supportive care.

# Contraindications

Recent studies conclude that acupuncture is a safe intervention for the general population, with minor adverse effects such as pain, slight bleeding, and bruising at needling sites, localized skin irritations, tiredness, and drowsiness (National Cancer Institute 2005). Cancer is not a contraindication for acupuncture treatment and eminent cancer organizations throughout the world support its use in supportive and palliative care (National Cancer Institute 2005, The Cancer Council Australia 2005). Patients seeking acupuncture treatment should ensure that the practitioner is appropriately qualified and registered. They should also understand fully that acupuncture treatment does not aim to cure cancer but may assist in the management of symptoms and side effects, as well as improve overall well-being.

Certain precautions should be observed, especially in frail and vulnerable patients who may be more sensitive to acupuncture. Strict clean needle technique is advised for patients who are immunocompromised (National Cancer Institute 2005). Needling should be avoided in the local area of an unstable spine, in tumour nodules and ulceration, in lymphoedematous limbs, in instances of severely impaired blood clotting, into a prosthesis, and in intracranial deficits (Tavares 2003).

It may be advisable for people with cancer seeking acupuncture treatment to find a practitioner who understands and has experience of working with cancer, its treatments, their side effects, and the signs of the progress of the disease.

## What happens during consultation and treatment?

As noted above, there are many different styles of acupuncture and the specifics of consultation and treatment vary accordingly. However, the following description is fairly typical of traditional acupuncture.

### Consultation

The first appointment with a traditional acupuncturist focuses on a full consultation. The practitioner gathers information about the main complaint(s), the patient's medical and family history, lifestyle, and circumstances, including emotions. The 'Ten Questions' are a traditional feature of the consultation and investigate aspects of the patient's life, including sleep patterns, food and taste, thirst and drink, bowels and urination, sweating, temperature preferences, head and body, eyes and ears, thorax and abdomen, and pain, with an additional category for health issues specific to women. The practitioner records the patient's pulse and may examine the tongue. The acupuncturist then interprets the collected information according to the principles of Chinese medicine, to devise the overall treatment principles appropriate for rebalancing the patient's *qi*. From this, the appropriate acupuncture points and treatment strategies are derived.

### Treatment planning

The acupuncturist and patient discuss the priority areas for treatment and the acupuncturist advises on the appropriate frequency of treatment and its expected duration. This will vary according to the nature of the condition, and its duration, as well as the patient's response to acupuncture. As a general rule, acute conditions respond more quickly, while chronic (long-standing) conditions may require prolonged treatment.

In the West, it is usual for patients to attend for treatment once or twice weekly initially. Sessions normally becomes less frequent as the condition improves and 'top-up' treatments may become the norm.

## Treatment

At each treatment, the acupuncturist will take the pulse and may examine the tongue and then insert needles into the appropriate acupuncture points. Acupuncture needles are very fine, solid needles usually made of stainless steel, very different from the hollow needles used for injections and blood tests. They are sterile and discarded after a single use. They are usually inserted superficially under the skin and then manipulated to obtain *deqi* or needle sensation. This is often described as being like a dull ache, or a tingling sensation, and is not intrinsically painful. Depending on the style of acupuncture, or the aims of the treatment strategy, the needles may be removed immediately after insertion or they may be left in place, typically for about 20 minutes.

During treatment, patients often experience a pleasant relaxed sensation or a feeling of heaviness in the limbs and some fall asleep. They may notice an immediate change in their symptoms after treatment or changes may take place gradually over time. Some change usually becomes apparent after three to five treatments. In addition to monitoring changes in their main symptoms, patients should look for changes in areas such as quality of sleep, levels of energy, and overall sense of well-being.

## Moxibustion

Moxibustion may be used during the treatment to warm, move, or nourish the *qi*. The dried herb, referred to as moxa, can be applied in a variety of ways. The practitioner may use a moxa stick, which is rather like a cigar. The glowing end of the lit stick is held above a point or moved back and forth over a channel or painful area to gently warm the area. Sometimes, a piece of moxa stick is applied to the handle of the needle and it infuses the acupuncture point with warmth. Small pieces of loose moxa may be rolled and placed directly on the acupuncture point and then lit with an incense stick to smoulder down. The moxa is removed as soon as the patient feels the warmth and the process repeated as appropriate. Acupuncturists take great care with moxa to ensure that the patient is never burned. As with acupuncture needling, many patients find moxa a relaxing and comforting form of treatment.

There are few studies investigating the use of moxibustion in the management of cancer but clinical observations indicate that it may be useful. Oncologists in a Beijing hospital find moxibustion is useful in treating immunodeficiency, leukopenia, squamous cell carcinoma, and other conditions (Peiwen 2003), whereas Japanese clinicians report that moxibustion is useful in the management and prevention of lymphoedema (National Cancer Institute 2005). Staebler (2006) advocates daily treatment with moxibustion for patients undergoing chemotherapy to counteract bone marrow suppression and teaches their carers to administer a simple protocol at home.

## Conclusion

Acupuncture can be used in conjunction with conventional cancer treatments and may be used at any stage of a person's cancer experience. Many individuals find acupuncture a beneficial treatment that can help manage cancer symptoms and treatment side effects. It can help patients, and their carers, to manage stress, cope with life, and improve their overall emotional and physical well-being. As one woman on a trial for using acupuncture to manage hot flushes said: 'I would recommend acupuncture as my quality of life was much improved as a result' (de Valois 2006*b*).

### Case study

'April' participated in a research study examining the use of ear acupuncture to manage the hot flushes and night sweats that are a common side effect of hormonal treatments in women with early breast cancer. She received ear acupuncture once a week for 8 weeks and was monitored for 30 weeks.

### Background

April, age 57, had been treated with surgery, chemotherapy, and radiotherapy and the last of these treatments had been 8 months prior to joining the ear acupuncture study. She had taken hormone replacement therapy for 5 years prior to her breast cancer diagnosis. She had been taking tamoxifen for 11 months and began to experience hot flushes soon after starting this. Feeling uncomfortable, out of control, and 'cross', April asked her consultant to change her medication. He suggested she try acupuncture.

On joining the study, April was experiencing an average of 12 flushing incidents per 24-hour period, with a range from 10–15 per day. Night sweats woke her three to four times per night and she found it difficult to get back to sleep. She had felt 'exhausted and wiped out' after chemotherapy. She did not feel she was getting much better although she followed a programme of regular gentle exercise to rebuild her strength gradually. Emotionally, she felt angry and frustrated; she was not as strong as before and could no longer do the same things. Her eyes felt dry and one would 'weep' when she got anxious.

### Progress through treatment

April reported that she felt very tired after the initial two ear acupuncture sessions. She found she needed a lot of sleep; but after the second treatment, she reported improvements in her quality of sleep. She also felt calmer in herself and had 'a feeling of well-being throughout the week'. The hot flushes were also becoming less frequent. At her fifth treatment, she noted that her energy was 'quite good', that her levels of flushing were staying constant in spite of warm weather, and she was feeling 'content and quite relaxed'. A week later, she reported that she was having much less trouble with her eyes. The following week, she was delighted to report that her husband had noticed that she had much more energy. At her eighth and final acupuncture session, April felt she had achieved her objectives: her hot flushes had reduced during the day, the night sweats had reduced in frequency and intensity, and she had a more peaceful sleeping pattern and improved levels of energy. She was also pleased that her eye problems had diminished.

## Long-term feedback

Four weeks after the end of her course of treatment, April wrote that she had been feeling 'more confident, more energetic, less tired because I have slept well at night. My dry eyes have improved a great deal'. At 18 weeks after the end of treatment, April still felt positive about her experience. She reported that her hot flushes were still not as intense as they had been. She also appreciated the opportunity to talk about her experience of breast cancer. Overall, she said that, during the course of acupuncture, she 'felt terrific—cheerful and full of energy ... I felt better physically' (de Valois 2006a).

# References

Birch, S. & Felt, R. L. 1999, *Understanding acupuncture*. Churchill Livingstone, Edinburgh.

de Valois, B. 2006a, Serenity, patience, wisdom, courage, acceptance: reflections on the NADA protocol, *European Journal of Oriental Medicine*, vol. 5, no. 3, pp. 44–9.

de Valois, B. 2006b, *Using acupuncture to manage hot flushes and night sweats in women taking tamoxifen for early breast cancer: two observational studies*. PhD thesis, Centre for Complementary Healthcare and Integrated Medicine, Thames Valley University.

Hicks, A., Hicks, J. & Mole, P. 2004, *Five element constitutional acupuncture*. Churchill Livingstone, Edinburgh.

House of Lords Select Committee on Science and Technology 2000, *Sixth report - complementary and alternative medicine (CAM)*, available at <http://www.parliament. the-stationery-office.co.uk/pa/ld199900/ldselect/ldsctech/123/12301.htm> (accessed November 22, 2005).

National Cancer Institute 2005, *Acupuncture (PDQ®): complementary and alternative medicine - health professional version*, available at <http://www.cancer.gov/cancertopics/ pdq/cam/acupuncture/HealthProfessional> (accessed October 6, 2006).

National Center for Complementary and Alternative Medicine 2004, *Acupuncture*, available at <http://nccam.nih.gov/health/acupuncture/> (accessed November 22, 2006).

National Institutes of Health 1997, *Acupuncture. NIH consensus statement online 1997 Nov 3–5 15(5)*, available at <http://consensus.nih.gov/1997/1997Acupuncture107html.htm> (accessed October 6, 2006).

Pan, C. X., Morrison, R. S., Ness, J., Fugh-Berman, A. & Leipzig, R. M. 2000, Complementary and alternative medicine in the management of pain, dyspnea, and nausea and vomiting near the end of life: a systematic review, *Journal of Pain and Symptom Management*, vol. 20, pp. 374–87.

Peiwen, L. 2003, *Management of Cancer with Chinese Medicine*. Donical Publishing Ltd, London.

Smith, J., Richardson, J., Filshie, J., Thomas, R., Moir, F. & Pilkington, K. 2005, *Acupuncture for hot flushes as a result of cancer treatment: a systematic review*, available at <http://rccm.org.uk/cameol/Default.aspx> (accessed October 18, 2005).

Staebler, F. 2006, The role of acupuncture and moxibustion in the treatment of cancer: part 2, *European Journal of Oriental Medicine*, vol. 5, no. 2, pp. 34–43.

Tavares, M. 2003, *National guidelines for the use of complementary therapies in supportive and palliative care*. Prince of Wales Foundation for Integrated Health, London.

The Cancer Council Australia 2005, *Position statement: complementary and alternative medicines*, available at <http://www.cancer.org.au/documents/Pos_Statem_Complementary_alternative_therapies_JUN05.pdf> (accessed November 21, 2006).

World Health Organisation 2003, *Traditional medicine*, available at <http://www.who.int/gb/ebwha/pdf_files/WHA56/ea5618.pdf> (accessed October 2, 2006).

Chapter 9

# Aromatherapy

Jacqui Stringer

## Summary

Aromatherapy uses essential oils derived from plants to enhance psychological and/or physical well-being. In the cancer care setting, it is often used to help reduce emotional distress and improve quality of life. Certain oils play a role in managing skin infections, inflammation, and lesions caused by the disease or its treatment. Aromatherapy in this setting must be adapted for patients' individual needs and vulnerabilities and there are important safety considerations.

## What are essential oils?

Essential oils are chemical compounds produced by plants. They have wonderful qualities including aromas that can evoke powerful memories, lift the spirit, and neutralize malodours. Some have analgesic, anti-inflammatory, or anti-microbial properties. Each plant produces its own essential oil and essential oils can be claimed as 'pure' only if they have been derived from the same plant source. Not all plants produce essential oils—those that do are called aromatics and include herbs (e.g. rosemary), flowers (e.g. rose), and trees (e.g. rosewood). Essential oils may be responsible for a number of activities within the plant, the main ones being attraction (of pollinators), repulsion (of predators), and protection (against infection). Essential oils are held in different parts of the plant; for example, the oil of flowering plants such as rose, chamomile, or jasmine is found in the flowers themselves, whereas that of herbs such as rosemary, basil, or bay is found in the leaves. Other sections of plants that may contain essential oils include resin, roots, and fruit. As the oil is housed in different areas of the plant, it can be harvested in different ways (e.g. expression, distillation, and solvent extraction).

## Modes of action

### Physiological

Depending on the essential oils used by a therapist and the manner in which they are administered, the mode of action will vary (Lis-Balchin 2006). The different chemical components of individual oils impact on the body in different ways, partly dependent on the manner in which they are used (e.g. orally, inhaled, or rectally). This chapter focuses mainly on dermal application within the context of an aromatherapy massage. Following such a massage, many of the chemical components of essential oils will be absorbed into the epidermis and dermis and through these into the bloodstream. Theoretically, this means that they are able to impact physiologically on bodily organs. Realistically, because of the low concentrations of oils used (commonly around 1%), it is unlikely that they would have any substantial influence—although clinical studies to validate this statement are not currently available. The only exception to be envisaged would be the use of oils for topical conditions such as reactions to drugs or cutaneous infections.

### Psychological

Because of the direct access of aromatic molecules to the brain through the olfactory membrane of the nasal passages, the potential for psychological impact—through, for example, memories triggered within the limbic system—is far greater than that for physiological change within this setting. However, because of the individualistic nature of memory, it is difficult to predetermine a person's response to a particular aroma—it will depend on the hedonic quality (perceived pleasantness/unpleasantness) of the odour for that individual.

## Definition and history

Aromatherapy is the practice of using volatile plant oils, primarily essential oils, either on their own or as part of another therapy (e.g. massage), to enhance psychological and/or physical well-being of the client.

Essential oils have been in use for thousands of years; Mary is said to have anointed the feet of Christ with oil of spikenard to give him spiritual strength prior to his crucifixion and the ancient Egyptians used oils such as cedarwood, cinnamon, and myrrh to embalm the dead.

During the early 1900s, a French perfumer and chemist named Gattefossé began exploring the medicinal use of essential oils—after burning his arm in his laboratory, he immersed it in a vat of lavender oil, which was the closest liquid to hand, and the burn healed rapidly with minimal scarring.

Gattefossé is credited with inventing the term 'aromatherapy'. Aromatherapy has gradually become more popular since the late 1900s and today it is one of the most widely used complementary therapies within the cancer care setting.

One of the benefits of integrating the use of essential oils into the care of the patient with cancer is that under certain circumstances they offer effective alternatives to the constant stream of drugs used to help alleviate symptoms of the disease and side effects of treatment. Some patients feel most comfortable using conventional medicine for problems such as mucositis, anxiety, or nausea. Many, however, express a desire to reduce their intake of drugs and in some cases this has proved possible by using essential oils in novel but appropriate ways. For example, abdominal massage using essential oils has been used to prevent constipation and essential oils as an adjunct to massage help alleviate anxiety.

When thinking about enhancing quality of life for patients with cancer, topics such as stress relief, improved sleep, reduction of anxiety, and enhanced body image are of primary importance. The most common way of utilizing essential oils in this area of clinical care is in conjunction with massage.

## Case 1

Kathryn was a ward sister diagnosed with acute lymphoblastic leukaemia. She failed to go into remission initially but eventually her leukaemia was brought under control and she received a matched unrelated donor transplant. This was the beginning of a very distressing stream of complications including life-threatening viral infections (through which she lost her sight almost completely), graft-versus-host disease, and severe mucositis. Through much of the next year, she fluctuated between being withdrawn and openly distressed as she watched her body fade away and her legs and feet swell with accumulation of oedematous fluid. Kathryn was by nature a reserved person who did not feel comfortable discussing her concerns with the medical team—she would always tell them she was 'fine' even when she obviously was not. Soon after her initial diagnosis, Kathryn became interested in aromatherapy massage and she found a window of relief through this in whatever problems she encountered. She very rarely talked during her sessions; in fact, she was often asleep by the end of the 20 minutes. One session, which particularly indicates how significant the massage was to her, was given on the day she passed away. Due to a viral infection, her breathing was laboured, her oxygen saturations were very low, and she was visibly distressed. The look of relief on her face when I entered the room was heart-warming. With a blend of lavender and rose (her favourite oils), I used gentle holding techniques on her feet, hoping to ground her and reduce her anxiety. By the end of the session, her breathing was calm and even, her saturations increased, and she was asleep. She died a few hours later. To ease someone's passing in such a way is both an honour and a blessing.

## Aromatherapy massage

Full-body massages are not appropriate for patients undergoing active cancer treatment; far from relaxing them, they are likely to exhaust them. Furthermore, patients undergoing chemotherapy are often hypersensitive to touch, so a prolonged massage would become irritating. What is appropriate is for patients to choose which part of the body they would like worked on, depending on areas of discomfort; this ensures that the patient obtains physical relief and also maintains control of the session. Ways in which sessions can be standardized to ensure safe practice include the time spent (20 minutes) on each massage and the type of strokes used (mainly light effleurage/stroking movements). The 20-minute guideline is not arbitrary; it is based on research suggesting that 15–20 minutes is sufficient to impact on various aspects of emotional distress, while avoiding over-stimulation of hypersensitive skin. With regard to technique, it must be explained to the patient before the session begins that deep massage movements (such as deep tissue kneading) are inappropriate while they are undergoing medical treatment and could even be counter-productive. Chemotherapy often induces some level of myelosuppression and so deep massage may cause bruising or a petechial rash in the thrombocytopenic patient.

## Research on the benefits of essential oils

To date, relatively few researchers have tried to evaluate the benefits of using essential oils in association with massage to improve the quality of life of patients with cancer (Corner 1995). However, Kite *et al.* (1998) in an evaluation of their service at a cancer support centre confirmed the role played by aromatherapy massage in reducing psychological distress. Wilkinson *et al.* (1999), working in a hospice setting, suggested that the benefits of massage are greater when essential oils are used, although not necessarily to the point of statistical significance. Fellowes *et al.* (2004), in a review of clinical trials on the topic of massage and aromatherapy for patients with cancer, concluded that evidence was mixed as to whether the use of essential oils enhanced the benefits seen from massage in patients with cancer. Unfortunately, the studies identified had used a maximum of two essential oils, but more commonly only one. The concern with this approach is that it only assesses the benefits of individual oils, rather than the benefits of aromatherapy in which several oils are usually used in combination. In an attempt to understand what receiving aromatherapy massage meant to patients with cancer, Dunwoody *et al.* (2002) explored the qualitative aspects of receiving massage. In this study, aromatherapy massage was carried out in a clinically appropriate manner, with both the therapist and the patient choosing the oils for the massage. The results confirmed the de-stressing effects of massage, in addition to highlighting other benefits such as empowerment of the patient.

## Adaptations for the cancer care setting

As with all touch therapy techniques used in the cancer care setting, practitioners need to be mindful that adaptations will be required in the use of essential oils.

### Concentration of oils

Patients undergoing treatment for cancer often have deranged serum biochemistry, suggesting that vital organs such as the liver and kidneys are under strain through the increased workload of metabolizing drugs. Consequently, it is inappropriate to use high concentrations of oils in this setting. For quality of life indications such as anxiety or depression, a 1% concentration is appropriate; this is strong enough to impact on the olfactory system but not to have a clinically relevant impact on the workload of the liver and kidneys. Using low concentrations of oils, there need be no concern over patients using the oil blend on a daily basis if they find it beneficial—as long as they adhere to the principle of choosing only one part of the body to be massaged. However, for patients with severely deranged liver or kidney function, it is better to explore alternative methods of delivery; for example, vaporizing oils during the massage but using only carrier oil on the skin.

### Aroma sensitivity

Just as patients may be hypersensitive to touch, they are also predisposed to taste change, sensitivity to smells, and change in odour preferences. Therefore, therapists need to be mindful that intense smells will be overwhelming and partiality to certain aromas may change frequently—particularly in the nauseated patient. For this reason, patients will often prefer oils with high tones, such as citrus oils. Oils that linger, such as patchouli or rose, should be used in moderation.

### Blending oils

Another concern associated with the concept of aroma sensitivity is that patients may become conditioned to certain odours. The patient is then at risk of associating a certain smell with a certain outcome. For example, if the patient was feeling nauseated while smelling a particular aroma, they are at risk of feeling nauseated every time they smell it in the future. One way to manage this is to ensure that patients only receive therapy with blended oils; although they may come across the smell of lavender, for example, outside the environment of their therapy, it is unlikely they will encounter the aroma of lavender blended with frankincense and thus the feeling of nausea will not be triggered.

## Oestrogenic oils

Traditionally, there have been concerns regarding the use of certain oils within the field of cancer care, specifically those with oestrogen-like components for patients suffering from oestrogen-dependent cancers (ovarian, breast, and uterine). The reality is that if the preceding guidelines relating to concentration of oils, blending oils, and length of massage are followed, then the impact of such oils is highly unlikely to be clinically relevant. However, because alternative oils with similar properties but without the oestrogenic components are always available, it is prudent to avoid those known to have such constituents until there is concrete evidence of their safety. Commonly used oils that need to be avoided in these patients include aniseed, fennel, clary sage, and niaouli. Two very useful oils over which concern is often voiced are rose and geranium. There is no clear evidence that such concerns are valid and in light of their obvious clinical benefits, it is not felt necessary to exclude them from practice.

## Antimicrobial action

So far, we have explored the use of essential oils in relation to enhancing patients' well-being through augmenting the relaxation effect of massage. However, essential oils possess many other useful qualities. For example, different oils are recognized as antimicrobial agents (Mishra and Dubey 1994; Gravett 2001), anti-inflammatory agents, and expectorants (Price and Price 1999). The antimicrobiological effects, which have been confirmed in both laboratory and clinical studies, are illustrated by the cases below.

---

### Case 2

Tim was 21 and suffering from acute leukaemia. He enjoyed his regular aromatherapy massages, saying they gave him the strength to cope with both his illness and the high-dose chemotherapy necessary to treat it. Unfortunately, his bone marrow took longer and longer to reconstitute after each course of treatment, leaving him vulnerable to infection during this time. It was anticipated that his treatment would culminate in a bone marrow transplant to give him the best chance of cure. During his penultimate course of chemotherapy, a scan showed a large fungal mass in his lungs—an aspergilloma. At this point, treatment was stopped and he was sent home on oral antifungal treatment only—to be married and for palliative follow-up only. He and his fiancée, as well as the staff on the unit, expected his marriage to be a short one.
It was suggested to Tim that he take home a bottle of blended essential oils with known antifungal properties to use in an inhalation three times daily along with his standard antifungal drugs. Tim came back for a repeat scan 4 months later; his chest was clear and he went on to receive a transplant.

### Case 3

Penny was a middle-aged woman being treated for multiple myeloma. Unfortunately, due to the ensuing neutropaenia, she contracted several very painful vulval lesions that were found to be infected with pseudomonas and proved to be resistant to antibiotics. A 3% blend of oils known to be active against pseudomonas was made up into an aqueous gel and applied to the lesions three times daily. Within 2 weeks, the lesions had healed.

It is important to remember that innovations that have been successful in individual cases such as the preceding ones need to be carefully thought out and validated through research before being widely used. Equally, data is urgently required relating to the biochemical effects of the oils—do they interact with chemotherapy, influence blood biochemistry, or vary the dosage of drugs received by a patient through binding to specific proteins?

## Other potential benefits

Essential oils have the potential to help in managing a number of other clinical problems, examples of which are given below.

### Reduced skin integrity

All forms of cancer treatment have the potential to impact negatively on the condition of the skin, through, for example, surgical wounds, burning and inflammation from radiation, or dryness after chemotherapy. Certain oils, combined with an appropriate carrier medium, can help in these situations. Lavender, for example, is well recognized for treating reduced skin integrity. Oils with recognized anti-inflammatory properties, such as yarrow or chamomile, can be used in cases of skin irritation.

### Fungating wounds

Fungating wounds are very distressing to both patients and their carers. These lesions are progressive, unsightly, and often malodorous. They cause misery to the patients who feel they are repulsive to others and upset the carers, who are worried that their aversion may be obvious to their loved ones. In addition to their inherent malodour, such lesions are a prime site for secondary bacterial infections that compound the problem. Essential oils applied in a suitable carrier (e.g. water-based gel) can be very useful in such situations; not only do they neutralize the malodour (rather than masking it) but oils with antimicrobial action (such as lavender or palma rosa) will also help protect against secondary infection.

### Wound care

Wounds caused by surgery for cancer may require a long time to heal, particularly if chemotherapy was given beforehand. Essential oils can be very useful in this arena. Their wound-healing properties have been recognized for thousands of years; frankincense and myrrh were held to be of equivalent value to gold at the time of Christ for their healing capacity, both physical and spiritual, and are still accepted in those terms today.

---

### Case 4

Martin, 18 years old, had been battling the effects of Crohn's disease for years. One of the issues he had to deal with was that once the integrity of his skin was broken it took many months to heal—sometimes up to a year. Surgery some weeks previously had left him with a long, deep wound in his upper thigh, which not only refused to heal but also kept him in a state of constant pain; having the wound dressed was excruciating and required him to be given both morphine and entanox. Following the complete breakdown of the wound site, there was a request for aromatherapy support. A 3% mix, which included palma rosa and geranium, was blended in a water-based gel and applied daily. Within 2 weeks, the wound was all but healed.

---

## Anxiety and panic attacks

For acute episodes of anxiety or panic, essential oils can be used in ways other than in massage. One very effective method is simple inhalation—putting a drop of oil (e.g. neroli) onto a tissue paper and encouraging the patient to take deep breaths. If there is the opportunity for massage, then so much the better; a foot massage will help ground the person—anchoring them back into their body. If this is done with essential oils blended into the carrier, then the same blend can be offered to the patient to take away with them, both to reinforce the feeling of calm and to inhale if they become overwhelmed once again.

## Safety issues

Although essential oils have much to offer within the sphere of cancer care, there are also a number of issues to be mindful of to ensure safe practice. Some of the concerns have been dealt with in detail in this chapter, while others have not. The main issues are listed below but it is important to note that this list is not exhaustive.

### Allergies/sensitivities

Patients may have pre-existing sensitivities or new ones that have been triggered by their recent treatments. It is imperative, therefore, that a thorough history be taken before therapy is initiated and, if appropriate, a patch test carried out.

### Deranged biochemistry

Liver or kidney function may be impaired through either medical treatment or disease status. Before using oils on the body, therefore, an assessment of organ function is required.

### Conditioned responses to oils

Conditioning to aromas can occur even after single pairings of a fragrance and a negative outcome (e.g. vomiting). This is particularly likely if the odour is a distinctive one and can lead to patients vomiting or feeling nauseated through smelling the oil or blend again.

## Concentrations of oils

In cancer care, it is suggested that a 1% concentration is appropriate for relaxation and for many skin-related concerns, particularly inflammatory conditions. It may be necessary to increase this slightly for specific situations such as topical applications for infection.

## Choice of oils

There are a few oils that are inappropriate in this field; also, it is critical to choose oils that are not overwhelming to the patient.

## Therapist qualifications

Because of the vulnerability of this client group, it is essential that therapists be qualified and insured with a recognized professional body. If they do not have prior experience of working in oncology, it is suggested they be supervised for a recommended period of 2 years by a senior therapist who has this experience.

# Documentation

♦ *Policies and guidelines*: These are necessary for therapists using essential oils in this environment. It is imperative that clear guidance be available for all therapists regarding all clinical issues. Therapists require a thorough understanding of cancer, its various treatments and side-effects, as well as the physiological and psychological impacts these have on patients

♦ *Consent form*: Confirming that the medical team is happy for a patient to be treated with essential oils when they are undergoing active treatment for cancer is necessary for each new referral

♦ *Treatment record*: This is maintained in order to record the patients' history, informed consent, and treatment sessions—including response. There are now publications that offer sample copies of referral and treatment records (Tavares 2003)

# Summary of recommendations

♦ Short (20-minute) massage sessions
♦ Low concentrations of essential oils (maximum of 1% for massage)
♦ When using essential oils, always follow up the session to ensure there have been no negative effects (e.g. sensitivities or conditioned reactions)

- Record all treatments appropriately; if essential oils have been used as part of a patient's clinical care, then this should be recorded in their clinical notes
- Develop practice slowly—integrate developments one at a time, using audit and evaluation to confirm outcomes and ensure best practice
- Choice of oils and any development of practice should be based on evidence—either your own or from good-quality research

## References

Corner, J., Cawley, N. & Hildebrand, S. 1995, An evaluation of the use of massage and essential oils on the well-being of cancer patients, *International Journal of Palliative Nursing*, vol. 1, no. 2, pp. 67–73.

Dunwoody, L., Smyth, A. & Davidson, R. 2002, Cancer patients' experiences and evaluations of aromatherapy massage in palliative care, *International Journal of Palliative Nursing*, vol. 8, no. 10, pp. 497–504.

Fellowes, D., Barnes, K. & Wilkinson, S. 2004, Aromatherapy and massage for symptom relief in patients with cancer (Cochrane Review), *The Cochrane Library*, Issue no. 3, pp. 1–19.

Gravett, P. 2001, Aromatherapy treatment for patients with Hickman line infections following high dose chemotherapy, *International Journal of Aromatherapy*, vol. 11, no. 1, pp. 18–19.

Hernandez-Reif, M., Field, T., Largie, S., Hart, S., Redzepi, M., Nierenberg, B. & Peck, M. 2001, Childrens' distress during burn treatment is reduced by massage therapy, *Journal of Burn Care Rehabilitation*, vol. 22, pp. 191–95.

Kite, S. M., Maher, E. J., Anderson, K. *et al.* (1998). Development of an aromatherapy service at a cancer centre, *Palliative Medicine*, vol. 12, pp. 171–80.

Lis-Balchin, M. 2006, *Aromatherapy Science*, a guide for healthcare professionals. Pharmaceutical Press.

Mishra, A. K. & Dubey, N. K. 1994, Evaluation of some essential oils for their toxicity against fungi causing deterioration of stored food commodities, *Applied and Environmental Microbiology*, vol. 60, pp. 1101–05.

Price, S. & Price, L. 1999, *Aromatherapy for health professionals*, Churchill Livingstone, Edinburgh.

Tavares, M. 2003, *National guidelines for the use of complementary therapies in supportive and palliative care*, The Prince of Wales' Foundation for Integrated Health, London.

Wilkinson, S., Aldridge, J., Salmon, I., Cain, E. & Wilson, B. 1999, An evaluation of aromatherapy in palliative care, *Palliative Medicine*, vol. 13, pp. 409–17.

## Reading list

Buckle, J. 2006, *Clinical Aromatherapy, Essential Oils in Practice.* 2nd edition. Churchill Livingstone, New York

Cancer Bacup Publications (website: www.cancerbacup.org.uk)

Chapter 10

# Art therapy

Paola Luzzatto and Bonnie Gabriel

## Summary

In this chapter, we offer a definition of art therapy and a brief history of its development as a profession, first in the UK and USA, and then throughout the world. The main feature of art therapy is the use of images and imagination, through which patients can express, understand, and elaborate their emotions at a symbolic level, within the therapeutic relationship. We describe some basic interventions for complementary and palliative care: bedside interventions with hospitalized patients, the open studio with patients during treatment, and group and individual art therapy.

## Definition

Art therapy is a form of psychotherapy that uses both verbal and non-verbal communication. The specificity of art therapy is based on its tri-polar setting, with the patient, the therapist, and the image as the three poles of a triangle. Within this specific setting, art therapy provides the possibility for patients to express, share, and transform their inner world through the dynamic use of images and imagination, within the therapeutic relationship with the art therapist.

## Brief history

Art therapy started in the 1940s and 1950s, in the UK and USA, as some artists started to work with war veterans and in psychiatric hospitals. During the 1960s and 1970s formal training was established, national associations were formed, and art therapists were employed in a variety of mental health institutions. In the UK, art therapy was recognized in 1982 as a distinct therapeutic modality by the National Health Service and in 1992 as a form of psychotherapy. Professional licensing to art therapists was approved in 2006 in New York State. Training courses have developed not only in most European countries but in many other parts of the world: Australia, Brazil, Canada, India, Israel, Mexico, Saudi Arabia, Singapore, South Africa, Taiwan, and Thailand.

In most countries, art therapy is now applied not only in psychiatric hospitals but also in educational and medical settings. Art therapy in complementary and palliative care started in paediatric settings and then expanded to treat adult patients with cancer. The Department of Psychiatry at Memorial Sloan-Kettering Cancer Center (MSKCC) in New York included art therapy in the psycho-oncology program for adult patients with cancer in 1995 (Luzzatto and Gabriel 1998). A variety of books on art therapy in complementary and palliative care have been published in the USA (Malchiodi 1998, 1999) and UK (Pratt and Wood 1998, Waller and Sibbett 2005). The first randomized, controlled study on the effectiveness of art therapy in psycho-oncology was recently conducted in Sweden (Oster *et al.* 2006) and represents an important landmark.

## The theory

The therapeutic factors in art therapy are based on the professional use of the triangular relationship between the patient, the image, and the therapist (Luzzatto 1989). Different communicative dimensions may be emphasized during the process—the patient may relate to the image, to the therapist, or to the therapist through the image. These dimensions may be used separately but they are always connected and affect each other (Fig. 10.1).

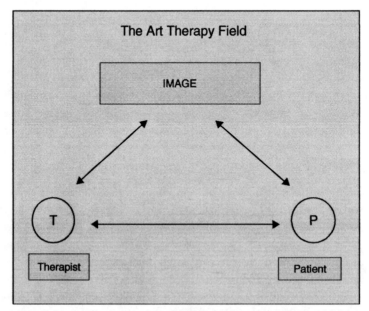

**Figure 10.1** The three communicative dimensions in the art therapy setting: (a) between the patient and the image; (b) between the patient and the therapist through the image; and (c) between the patient and the therapist.

The 10 factors listed below enable the art therapist in complementary and palliative care to deal with issues of pain, illness, and death. Art therapy can:

1. Facilitate a calm and positive mental state through the use of silence and concentration

2. Stimulate a sense of freedom and energy through cathartic and creative image making

3. Allow the expression of difficult feelings using non-verbal and symbolic communication

4. Offer safety through a double containment—the image and the art therapist

5. Strengthen self-identity through the process of distancing from the image and self-recognition

6. Allow the emerging of meaningful memories and thoughts following the flow of free associations

7. Stimulate group support and group interaction through non-verbal and verbal sharing and feedback

8. Help patients to reach self-understanding and insight through the dynamic use of images and imagination

9. Facilitate transformation of patients' feelings and thoughts through various creative techniques, within the relationship with the art therapist

10. Include the use of transference and counter-transference to facilitate the therapeutic process.

## Clinical interventions in complementary and palliative care

During 10 years of providing clinical art therapy at MSKCC, we have found some art therapy interventions particularly effective in responding to patients' needs. Here, we describe four of them: (1) bedside interventions for hospitalized patients; (2) the open studio during treatment; (3) The Creative Journey (short-term group art therapy); and (4) individual art psychotherapy.

### Bedside interventions

Patients may be in the hospital for just a few days (e.g. after surgery) or for several weeks (e.g. when undergoing bone marrow transplantation); in both cases, they are usually seen individually at the bedside. Sometimes, family groups may work together in the patient's room. Small sheets of paper and simple sets of art materials are recommended. If the patient feels inhibited by the white page, it may be useful to offer some guidance and facilitating techniques.

The art therapist may also work with the patient's environment; the view from the window and objects in the room may be starting points leading to a creative experience and symbolic self-expression. Patients at a terminal stage may not be able to hold a pen or a brush; the art therapist may paint for them, under their instructions. The art therapist can play a unique role in allowing patients to give form to their existential and spiritual needs. The study we have conducted with patients in isolation for bone marrow transplant (Gabriel *et al.* 2001) has shown that they may benefit from art therapy in a variety of ways: to feel more relaxed; to express and/or transform their state of mind; to communicate difficult sensations and feelings to relatives, friends, and medical staff; and to reflect on existential and spiritual issues.

## The drop-in open studio

Patients during treatment usually suffer from feelings of fatigue, anxiety, and distress and they welcome access to a supportive and flexible environment, which does not require regular attendance. A suitable art therapy intervention for these patients seems to be the drop-in open studio. Patients may come before or after treatments or medical appointments, engage in personal projects, and stay as long as they desire. A variety of art materials is readily available on the tables: white and colour paper, pencils, pastels, watercolour, tempera, and material for collage (magazines, scissors, and glue). Postcards and art books may also be stimulating for some patients. In the open studio, silence is encouraged and verbal interaction between patients is discouraged; nevertheless, the art therapist must be available to respond to patients who need to talk, without disrupting the quiet atmosphere of the room.

---

### Case 1

R, a young woman from Eastern Europe, comes to the art therapy open studio accompanied by a social worker. R had an appointment with her oncologist and was told she had a recurrence of breast cancer. She has a ticket to go back home but has been crying for a long time and expressed suicidal intentions, together with the wish of not returning home.

R sits at one of the small tables. She looks very withdrawn. I tell her she can choose a piece of paper of any colour and she selects black paper. I suggest she would place her hands on the paper and try to relax and breathe deeply, which she does. It looks as if she is appreciating the silence in the room and the presence of friendly people around her.

After a while, as R is very still, I suggest she might select a second piece of paper of a different colour. I add that she can do anything she wants with the two pieces of paper: draw or paint, or cut them into pieces. She chooses white paper this time and begins to cut it into pieces. One by one, she places them on the black paper. The white shapes on the black background look quite evocative. R continues to do her artwork, while I move around the room. When she finishes, she wants to tell me the meaning of each piece: 'this white strip is the floor, this is white milk spilled on the floor, this is a baby cot, and this is a blanket... this is a flower on the other side...' (Colour plate 1).

I ask whether she can give a title to her picture. She writes HOPE and then says her sister at home is expecting a baby. She wants to go home and see her. R looks surprised by her own work and is grateful for the experience: 'I have been talking and crying in the hospital all day… I have been here in this room for a long time, and I have never cried… I think I was not crying because I was not talking... And now this flower has appeared, and I know it means Hope… Thank you!' R takes her picture with her and leaves the room.

Comment: This patient was helped by a number of factors. She needed silence instead of words; she needed to distance herself from her immediate situation; she needed to get in touch with the creative and hopeful part of herself. The setting of the drop-in open studio offered what she needed. The following week, the social worker confirmed that R had been able to deal with her distress and together they made plans for her travels and her future treatment.

## Short-term group art therapy: The Creative Journey

Patients with cancer who have completed their treatment often feel vulnerable and ambivalent. The threat of a relapse is always a concern, which may become a reality. Patients may feel changed due to the cancer experience and may have to find a new identity and new meaning in their life. Often, this is the right time to commit to a weekly art therapy group.

There are many approaches to group art therapy, ranging from art-based workshops to psychoanalytically oriented groups. Another type that may be appropriate to patients with cancer is the theme-oriented art therapy group. The themes may be selected by the therapist or by the patients themselves and differ according to patients' needs. Themes may be closely related to their current concerns (coping with stress, facing loss, positive and negative relationships, etc.), based on reviewing and illustrating personal memories and life narratives or based on play and humour, imagination and fairy tales, dreams, contact with nature or spiritual needs, just to mention a few.

At MSKCC, we have created a 10-week group art therapy program called The Creative Journey, which seems particularly suited to patients with cancer (Luzzatto and Gabriel 2000). The aim is to help patients externalize and symbolize their inner world, which in turn helps them to strengthen their self-identity and deal with cancer-related issues. During each workshop, patients move through five stages: (1) a guided concentration; (2) a technique to facilitate image making (which is different each week); (3) the symbolization process; (4) distancing from the images; and (5) self-reflection, sharing, and feedback in the group. The 10 techniques of The Creative Journey facilitate the development of personal images in three ways: from the use of art materials, from external images, and from the inner world of the patients. The last workshop offers an opportunity to create an image that represents the patient's experience of The Creative Journey.

## Case 2

M is a 58-year-old woman who struggled with lung cancer for 8 years. Here is a list of the 10 workshops she attended of The Creative Journey, with the titles of her images and some of her comments and reflections.

1. Colours and shapes

   'Playing with fate'. M creates an image from origami paper cut into different shapes. The image contains a green field, pink angels, and blue sea waves. The green represents for her the natural world, the angels symbolize the world beyond, and the blue forms represent her cancer; she says the three elements are balanced.

2. Blind drawing

   'Table for two'. In using a scribble technique, M sees two figures threatened by a dark form but she feels supported by the relationship with her partner.

3. Self-introduction collage

   'The waterfall'. In the collage, there is a waterfall and a woman is standing calmly near it. M says that the turmoil is always there but one need not be caught in it.

4. Playing with art materials

   'The struggle'. An image of a bird emerges out of her playful use of colour pastels; the bird has a rope tied around its leg. M says that the image is a reflection of how she is feeling, now that she had just found out that her present treatment is no longer effective.

5. The hidden seed

   'Star-flower' (Colour plate 2). M draws a star-flower growing from a barren landscape, and she writes: 'Can a good seed grow in this landscape? ... Something meaningful may come from the most unexpected places ... if we remain engaged in the life process'.

6. Chaos and order

   'The golden space'. From the intentionally chaotic spread of colours, M selects a detail and develops it into a scene of a man and a woman in a protective golden space, under a red palm tree by the ocean, appreciating life while at the same time dealing with cancer.

7. The visual poem

   'Who knows?' M cuts a number of words from magazines and arranges them to make a poem. She says: 'These words speak about life and death'.

8. Stress and opposite

   'Balance'. M creates an image of two people on a seesaw. The seesaw rests on a triangle that symbolizes the strength of their relationship.

9. Still life and transformation

   'Connections'. M looks at a candle on the table and transforms it to create an abstract image, full of different colours. She says: 'The spiral of life goes on forever, and everything is connected'.

10. My creative journey

    'Beyond the beyond' (Colour plate 3). M makes a collage representing two swans and writes: 'In the storm I am, in the storm we are ... In the simplicity of all things I will be there for you'.

Comment: This patient had never painted before and found that through the image-making process she was able to access a part of herself that would be very difficult to verbalize. Her main theme was the process of separating from her relationship with her partner and from this world; she referred to it as the transition to the beyond. Through review of her images,

M was able to recount and hold on to many meaningful memories, accept the losses, and strengthen her spirituality. She felt that life had been good for her because she had been able to give and receive love.

## Individual art therapy

Individual art therapy offers a different therapeutic process to each patient. Some people with cancer need to process their experience of the illness; some to focus on their present life situation; others to face unresolved issues from the past. Some need to learn to be creative; others to channel their emotions in a positive way. Some need to learn how to live again; others how to accept death.

### Case 3

C is a woman in her thirties, diagnosed with melanoma with a poor prognosis. Her psychiatrist has referred her to art therapy in the hope that she can explore the reality of her situation within a different modality since she seems unable to talk about herself in the verbal encounters. Most of all, the psychiatrist is concerned that this patient has cut herself off from her 7-year-old daughter. She is divorced and has left her daughter with her own mother in Israel, as she is living in New York.

I saw C once a week for 6 months. She came to art therapy with great enthusiasm. Nevertheless, when she started to use art materials, she soon felt at a loss, unable to draw, paint, or 'imagine'. Together, we realized that she could not 'play' with art materials, maybe because she had not learned to play as a child. In this way, she got in touch with some of her early unfulfilled needs. This awareness helped her to think also of her daughter's needs.

When C started to work with the technique of collage, she never tired of cutting out beautiful landscapes and seascapes; she said these were all countries she wanted to visit in the future. Working through her wish to travel, C slowly started to make connections with the precariousness of her plans and with her emotions. Some sadness and concern emerged for herself, for her mother, and for her daughter.

One day, while working on a collage, she saw a picture about a Jewish festival. She talked to me about the Jewish religion and started to draw Jewish sacred objects, describing what each of them meant and how they were used during the rituals. For a while, each session became the story of a ritual and this task seemed to help her to move her attention from the material world to more abstract and existential meanings. Issues of life and death and of facing the unknown emerged almost naturally. At this point, she started to talk about her wish to go back to Israel, to say goodbye to her daughter and her family. She started to make regular telephone calls to her daughter and to send her little gifts. She was aware that she was alone in the face of death. She had become more capable of dealing with her emotions and with existential issues. Her initial grandiosity was leaving space to the awareness of life's limitations.

One day, she wanted to use brush and tempera for the first time. She painted an image of herself on the beach, sitting on the sand, looking at the immensity of the sea. She had always used pencil and pastels and now she felt happy about the fluidity of the art material. She loved the sensation of the brush and the tempera. The following week, she wanted to look again at the image she had painted of herself on the beach; we looked at it together in silence for some time.

She said: 'I like this picture. In this picture I am sitting on the sand, and I am looking at the sea…' I asked: 'And what do you see?' She took another piece of paper, and she slowly painted a series of arches on the water; each arch was of a different colour. She said: 'I am looking at this arch… it is a very special bridge—a bridge towards the unknown' (Colour plate 4).

Comment: The main aspect of this individual therapy was the patient's gradual development of symbolic thinking. She moved out from the concrete attention to her own illness to reach an appropriate concern for her daughter and was able to reconnect with her. In the end, this patient—who was at the beginning almost unable to imagine—made a deeply symbolic painting of a rainbow bridge on the sea and through this image she reached a peaceful awareness of moving towards the mysterious dimension of the unknown.

## Criteria for referral to art therapy

Which patients may benefit most from art therapy? From the literature, and from our experience at MSKCC, we suggest that most oncology patients may benefit at various stages of their illness: from the traumatic moment of diagnosis, to the exhausting period of treatment, to the difficult time of post-treatment, or during the terminal stage. The art therapy interventions must be modified to fit their changing needs.

When an art therapist is a member of a treatment team, other professionals may refer patients to art therapy. It is important to make sure patients know that an art therapy intervention is not an art class; the expression of the Self is at the core of art therapy and the revealing images that may emerge during sessions can be used to increase self-awareness and self-understanding.

Three categories of patients who may benefit in a special way from this approach are:

◆ Withdrawn and uncommunicative

◆ Showing anxious or depressed moods

◆ Searching for spiritual meaning in their life

It may be difficult to help these patients through talking or drugs alone and a referral to art therapy can add a new creative dimension to the treatment. The withdrawn patient may be helped by the symbolic indirect way of communicating. Sometimes, a very simple beginning is sufficient, like making a mark or a squiggle on the paper, and developing it slowly into an image; the image may be intriguing and surprising and lead to a verbal exchange with the art therapist and to a more meaningful communicative level.

Physical and psychological pain may be externalized and expressed visually through the symbolic use of colours, shapes, or images cut out from magazines and made into a collage (Luzzatto *et al.* 2003). The anxious and depressed patient may respond particularly well to art therapy interventions. The anxious patient may be able to relax, the depressed patient may feel energized, and they may also move into a deeper understanding of the factors behind the anxious or depressed state.

We have found that the symbolic process of image making can be particularly appropriate for patients who need to explore existential, spiritual, or religious issues and who find it difficult to share these concerns verbally with staff and relatives. Images from nature seem to be particularly helpful in dealing with the unknown and the infinite, reviewing one's life, and confronting death-related issues. The area of complementary and palliative care needs to move along the road of inter-disciplinarily work and reciprocal referral for the benefit of our patients.

## References

Gabriel, B., Bromberg, E., Vandenbovenkamp, J., Walka, P., Kornblith, A. B. & Luzzatto, P. 2001, Art Therapy with adult bone marrow transplant patients in isolation: a pilot study, *Psycho-Oncology*, vol. 10, pp. 114–23.

Luzzatto, P. 1989, The relationship between art and therapy, *Inscape: The Journal of the British Association of Art Therapy*, Autumn Issue, 31.

Luzzatto, P. & Gabriel, B. 1998, Art Psychotherapy, in ed. J. Holland, *Psycho-Oncology*. Oxford University Press, New York.

Luzzatto, P. & Gabriel, B. 2000, The Creative Journey: a model for short-term group art therapy with post-treatment cancer patients, *Art Therapy*, vol. 17, pp. 265–9.

Luzzatto, P., Sereno, V. & Capps, R. 2003, A communication tool for cancer patients with pain: the art therapy technique of the Body Outline, *Palliative and Supportive Care*, vol. 1, pp. 135–42.

Malchiodi, C. (ed) 1999a, *Art Therapy with Children*, Jessica Kingsley, London.

Malchiodi, C. (ed) 1999b, *Art Therapy with Adults*, Jessica Kingsley, London.

Oster, I., Svensk, A. C., Magnusson, E. *et al.* 2006, Art Therapy improves coping resources: a randomized, controlled study among women with breast cancer, *Palliative and Supportive Care*, vol. 4, pp. 57–64.

Pratt, M. & Wood, M. (eds) 1998, *Art Therapy in Palliative Care*, Routledge, London.

Waller, D. & Sibbett, C. (eds) 2005, *Art Therapy and Cancer Care*, Open University Press, New York.

## Organizations

American Art Therapy Association: email arttherapy@ntr.org; web site: www.arttherapy.org

British Association of Art Therapists: email baat@ukgateway.net; web site: www.baat.org

International Networking Group of Art Therapists email: art_tx@earthlink.net; web site: www.acteva.com/go/inga

Chapter 11

# Bach flower remedies

Jennifer Barraclough

## Summary

Bach flower remedies are a form of 'energy' or 'vibrational' medicine, focused on the emotional level. Besides the well-known combination Rescue™ Remedy, this system comprises 38 individual essences, mostly derived from plants and trees that grow wild in England and Wales. Discovered in the 1930s, these remedies have become popular all over the world as an aid to managing psychological distress, including that associated with cancer. Little formal research has been published but a descriptive account is provided in this chapter in the hope of encouraging further studies.

## Introduction

The Bach system is a good example of a holistic therapy. It treats the person and not the disease, considering each client as a unique individual rather than pre-scribing a standard treatment for certain symptoms or diagnoses. It encourages self-responsibility for healing, rather than being based on an authoritarian doctor–patient relationship. It is derived from nature, carries no risk of serious side effects, and can safely be combined with other treatments. Instead of dwelling only on what is wrong with people, it emphasizes the idea that illness can be a learning experience and even a transformative one.

Bach's remedies are used by millions of people all over the world and several similar systems using the native flowers of other countries have been developed as an off-shoot of his work. However, because of the lack of a scientific evidence base, few conventional healthcare professionals are prepared to take these remedies seriously. Coming from an orthodox medical background, I was also sceptical when I began studying the remedies out of curiosity, so the many excellent responses I observed when I administered them to my friends and family—many of them equally sceptical—truly surprised me. Having been convinced that there was something about the system that really worked,

I went on to train as a Bach Foundation Registered Practitioner and have since treated a number of clients suffering from cancer-related distress.

## Case 1

Margaret had been diagnosed with pulmonary metastases from breast cancer, 8 years after her primary treatment. She had had several episodes of acute psychiatric disturbance following adverse life events in the past but had experienced such severe side effects from various psychotropic drugs that she was unwilling to take any more of these and asked for a course of Bach flowers instead. As a person always highly sensitive to stress and change (*Walnut*), she was kept awake at night by worrying thoughts (*White Chestnut*) and described feelings of grief and shock (*Star of Bethlehem*), discouragement (*Gentian*), and anxiety about the prospect of further chemotherapy (*Mimulus*). She described the remedies as 'soft and fabulous' and reported that, along with the support from the local palliative care unit, they helped her cope with her situation. Two years later, her physical disease remained well controlled by medical treatment and she had maintained her mental equilibrium. However, she requested further remedies because of exhaustion following a course of manual lymphatic drainage and was given a single flower, *Olive*.

## Edward Bach MBBS, MRCS, LRCP, DPH

The life and work of Dr Edward Bach (pronounced Batch) is described here because it illustrates many principles of the holistic approach. Bach was born in 1886 into an English family of Welsh descent, studied medicine in Birmingham and London, and qualified from University College Hospital in 1912, 2 years before the start of the First World War. Frail since childhood, he was turned down for military service but undertook many extra duties such as caring for those wounded in war besides continuing in his post in the hospital. In 1917, aged 31, he suffered a 'collapse' attributed to overwork and had a severe haemorrhage. After abdominal surgery, he was diagnosed as having advanced cancer, with only about 3 months to live. In the hope of making a lasting contribution to medicine before he died, Bach threw himself back into work again and soon became stronger although he frequently stayed up all night in his laboratory. This experience convinced him that mental states could have a powerful influence on physical ones.

He continued working in London for several years, making good career progress in conventional terms: specializing in pathology and bacteriology, obtaining a Diploma in Public Health, holding posts in various London hospitals, and having private practice in Harley Street. However, he became increasingly disillusioned with orthodox medicine, believing that the treatments were too toxic and only 'dealing with results and not causes'. He wanted to find forms of natural healing that would treat the whole individual, rather than just symptoms and diseases. The study of homeopathy fulfilled this ideal to some extent and his research at the London Homeopathic Hospital led to the development of 'bowel nosodes'—bacterial preparations that became the basis of some homeopathic vaccines still used today. The new system of flower essences that Bach was soon to discover has much in common with homeopathy, although there are also important differences. Meanwhile, he was developing his philosophy of health and disease and a simple method of personality typing. He originally assumed that certain personality types would be prone to certain diseases. Later, he concluded this was not the case but believed that personality type would determine the individual's reaction to being ill and therefore indicate a starting point for treatment.

In 1928, while visiting Wales, Bach intuitively discovered his first two wild flower remedies: *Impatiens* for the impatient, irritable type of person and *Mimulus* for the anxious or phobic type. He soon found a third, *Clematis*, for the day-dreamer who is wrapped up in fantasies of the future rather than focusing on present reality. He achieved such good results with these three flower remedies that he soon abandoned all other forms of treatment.

In 1930, he left London, spending next the few years in Wales and Norfolk and walking hundreds of miles in search of more healing plants. This was an intensive and painful experience for him because he would be assailed by a negative emotion that continued until he found the flower with the right 'vibrations' to make him feel better again.

Around this time, Bach wrote a short book *Heal Thyself*, which has become a classic although much of the philosophy outlined in it is not original. In summary, although Bach acknowledged the importance of physical factors in both causation and treatment of disease, he believed the fundamental cause of most ill-health was 'a prolonged conflict between soul and personality' involving a departure from the sufferer's own true path in life and/or misguided attitudes towards others. Such errors would lead to an emotional imbalance that, in turn, would increase vulnerability to material pathogens. He regarded suffering, although apparently cruel, as a potential force for good because it enabled people to see their faults and overcome them.

It is important to understand that the flower remedies can be successfully used without any reference to these ideas. Although some people suffering from major medical conditions find them of great interest and relevance, others perceive them as distressing rather than helpful. Despite the many research studies carried out since Bach's time, the question of whether they are valid in relation to cancer is still unresolved.

Bach described a number of ways of maintaining or recovering good health: cultivation of virtues to replace faults, willingness to learn from all aspects of life, banishment of fear, practising care and respect for the physical body, becoming more open to intuitions from the higher self through meditation, and periods of rest and relaxation. 'For those who are sick, peace of mind and harmony with the soul are the greatest aid to recovery'. He advocated that 'We must plunge into life, developing our individuality in accordance with the Soul's direction, and love and help others without ever interfering with their own Soul path'.

In 1934, Bach moved to Mount Vernon, a cottage in the Oxfordshire village of Sotwell, with his devoted followers Nora Weeks and Victor Bullen. He found more remedies in the surrounding countryside, bringing the total to 38. The trio lived modestly, eating home-grown vegetables and using home-made furniture, for by this time Bach had used up or given away most of his money and possessions. His life was increasingly guided by the key value of simplicity. Indifferent to fame and fortune and conventional opinion, he treated patients free of charge. He saw masses of sick people and besides giving flower remedies, he had developed the gift of healing by touch alone. He carried on his work despite reprimands from the General Medical Council, which disapproved of his using unqualified assistants and advertising his talks in the local paper.

In 1935, Bach pronounced his life work complete. He said, 'This system of treatment is the most perfect which has been given to mankind within living memory' and asked that it be continued without distortion. The following year, aged 50, he died peacefully of 'heart failure' and was buried in the local churchyard. Nora and Victor stayed on at Mount Vernon and continued to practise and word of the flower remedies gradually spread further. Nora wrote a biography of Bach (Weeks 1940) on which the present summary is based. She died in 1978. Mount Vernon has been preserved as a charitable trust, the Dr Edward Bach Healing Trust, and is home to the Bach Centre (www.bachcentre.com).

Although the remedies are now made available on a large scale for worldwide distribution they are still prepared in the traditional manner, from flowers growing in their natural habitats and processed by Bach's original 'sun' or 'boiling' methods to extract their essence into water. The resulting fluid is diluted, preserved in brandy, and made up into the 'stock bottles' that are sold in health stores. Although the remedies can be taken in this concentrated form, it is more economical to dilute them into 'treatment bottles' according to the instructions given.

## Mode of action and efficacy

Anecdotal experience with thousands of cases for more than 70 years supports the benefits of the Bach flower remedies. However, their acceptance within orthodox medical circles has been understandably limited by two factors: the lack of well-designed clinical trials and the lack of any conventional scientific explanation for how they might work.

The remedies contain no detectable chemical extracts of their source plants but are said to carry their spiritual essence or energetic imprint, which corresponds on a vibrational level with positive qualities of mind or spirit. The therapeutic action comes from promoting these positive qualities, not from suppressing painful feelings or character flaws. For example, the effect of *Mimulus* would be to enhance courage rather than to mask fear. In Bach's words, the remedies work by 'flooding our bodies with the beautiful vibrations of our Higher Nature, in the presence of which disease melts away as snow in the sunshine'.

This bold statement is not to be taken too literally, for modern practitioners use the remedies for emotional disorders only and make no claim to the near-miraculous healings of physical conditions that Bach was apparently able to achieve for both his patients and himself.

At least 80% of clients treated by qualified practitioners report improvements in emotional state after taking the remedies, often describing quite striking and sustained responses. General factors—what some might call 'placebo response' but I prefer to call self-healing—undoubtedly contribute to this positive effect. This system encourages people to take responsibility by examining their situation from a new perspective and helping choose the flowers they need. I have had a few clients who for various reasons never actually took their remedies but improved all the same because the interview process had enabled them to approach their problems in a more constructive fashion.

There are also reasons to believe that the individual remedies do have specific effects. Animals and children often respond well, which suggests more than placebo. Some clients do not respond to one mixture but then improve with a different one. Others experience 'healing reactions' in the form of more intense emotions, vivid dreams, or mild physical symptoms such as skin rashes or loose bowel motions. Each remedy has a different profile on Kirlian photography and reacts differently in electro-acupuncture circuits.

Turning specifically to the cancer treatment setting, an audit from an oncology unit in the UK (Ann Hull, personal communication) described a series of 16 patients, many with advanced malignancies, who received four consultations over a 9-week period and were assessed before and after treatment with a widely used self-rating instrument, the Hospital Anxiety and Depression Scale. All of them had initially scored as probable psychiatric 'cases', with average scores of 17 for anxiety and 17 for depression (the maximum score on each scale is 21). At follow-up, all had improved substantially, with one patient still in the borderline case range but all the others in the normal range. Average scores were down to 3 for anxiety and 3 for depression. Many patients had been able to avoid taking psychotropic drugs or reduce their intake of these. Five years later, the service at this hospital continues to be funded, on an expanded scale, reflecting the high levels of satisfaction among patients, clinicians, and managers.

The few randomized clinical trials (RCTs) that have been carried out on defined populations (not including patients with cancer) do not confirm the impressive results seen in clinical practice and a systematic review (Ernst 2002) concluded that there is no evidence for anything more than a placebo response. However, most of these trials were flawed in that they involved giving set combinations of flowers for a particular condition, instead of individualized mixtures selected by personal interview, and achieved only low rates of follow-up. Nelsons, the firm of homeopathic manufacturers that prepares remedies for commercial sale, has recently carried out a more comprehensive review that includes qualitative studies as well as RCTs and has reached a more positive conclusion (Nelsons 2006). However, there is undoubtedly a need for better-designed studies to be carried out.

## Indications in the cancer care setting

To repeat, the remedies are not a treatment for the cancer itself and it is notable that no cancer cases are included in the book of clinical reports from the early days at Mount Vernon (Chancellor 1971), although this does gives many examples of recovery from physical disorders of a more 'functional' kind.

The remedies are, however, ideally suited to treatment of the emotional distress associated with cancer or any other serious disease. This ranges from the 'normal' situational reactions that affect the majority of patients at some stage to the more severe and prolonged psychiatric problems that develop in a minority. The remedies can also help with somatic symptoms in cases where psychological as well as physical factors are contributing.

---

### Case 2

Catherine, an elderly woman with a dual diagnosis of cancer and heart failure, was seen in her home because she was too weak and breathless to attend the clinic. She described feelings of desperation (*Sweet Chestnut*), hopelessness (*Gorse*), terror (*Rock Rose*), uncontrollable tearfulness (*Cherry Plum*), and guilt in case she had caused her illness through wrong attitudes or behaviour in the past (*Pine*). The day after starting the remedies, she phoned to say she felt far more 'calm and in control' and her breathing was so much better that she had walked to the shops. Her mental state continued to improve over the next few weeks.

---

Many of the other 38 flowers besides the ones already mentioned might be appropriate in the cancer care setting, for example, *Crab Apple* for body image problems and *Red Chestnut* for extreme concern about a loved one's welfare. Howard (2007) has discussed the role of the Bach remedies in the management of pain, including cancer pain.

## Contra-indications, precautions, and limitations

There is a theoretical possibility of ill-effects due to the alcohol content of the remedies. The stock bottles contain brandy as a preservative. By the time this concentrate has been diluted into a treatment mixture, the quantity of alcohol remaining is so tiny that the remedies are considered safe for pregnant women and babies. However, caution is required for three groups of people:

- ◆ Those with a past history of alcoholism
- ◆ Those taking prescribed drugs that interact with alcohol
- ◆ Those with moral or religious objections to alcohol

In such cases, it may be acceptable to apply the remedies to the skin or over the pulse points on wrists or temples.

The remedies have no side effects as such, but as mentioned earlier, they can cause 'healing reactions' with exacerbation of existing symptoms or emergence of new ones. Reactions are usually mild and transient and can be explained in terms of negative emotions being cleared from the system and therefore can be taken as a positive sign that the treatment is working. It is highly advisable to persevere in such cases, although it may be necessary to modify the mixture and a qualified practitioner can advise on this.

Because the selection of flowers depends entirely on the emotional state and personality of the individual and not on their medical diagnosis or physical symptoms, the approach to a patient with cancer is in one sense the same as for any other client. However, in order to relate appropriately to both patients and staff in the oncology setting, it would seem important for the practitioner to have at least a basic knowledge of the medical and psychosocial aspects of cancer and its management. In most cases, he or she would be well advised to focus the consultation simply on the way the patient is feeling at present, rather than raising the complex and sensitive question of whether psychological factors are important in the causation or progression of cancer. The practitioner also needs to be aware of his or her own emotional response to patients who are seriously ill and may be going to die. Independent supervision is highly desirable, especially for those without prior experience in this field.

The limitations of the Bach system must be kept in mind. In the setting of oncology and palliative care, the remedies would always need to be combined with other forms of treatment and support. In the words of the Bach Foundation's Code of Practice, 'practitioners shall confine themselves to commenting on and selecting remedies for perceived emotional states and personality types and shall not attempt to treat or diagnose for any physical or mental illness'.

## Levels of treatment

Treatment can be carried out at various levels of sophistication. The most widespread approach is by self-help, as encouraged by Bach himself. The remedies can be purchased from health stores in most countries and there are many excellent books explaining how to use them (e.g. Howard 1990; Ball 2003).

Healthcare professionals, including nurses and complementary therapists, who have undergone basic Bach flower courses may use the remedies as an adjunct to their main practice. For example, some nurses in oncology and palliative care like to offer flower remedies to their patients, although this practice is usually unofficial and unrecorded.

Bach Foundation Registered Practitioners have undergone a more extensive training comprising attendance at courses, essays, examinations, and written assessment of casework. A consultation with a qualified practitioner usually lasts about an hour. It begins with a brief explanation about the remedies and the practitioner may also give some information about Bach and his philosophy, although this is by no means always appropriate for patients who are very sick or distressed. The practitioner's aim is to understand the present emotional state, and perhaps the most prominent personality traits, but without probing too far beyond what is spontaneously revealed. The style of interview therefore tends to be friendly and conversational and less structured, detailed, or searching than that likely to be used by a mental health professional or a homeopath. Patients/clients are encouraged to take part in process of selecting their remedies if they wish.

The Bach Foundation does not support the use of special aids such as muscle testing or dowsing when selecting remedies. These methods are sometimes employed by therapists of other modalities but their validity is not established and they can have the significant disadvantage of by-passing the interview assessment, which is such an important part of the consultation process.

The most widely used preparation, certainly in the self-help field, is the Rescue™ Remedy. This is a combination of five flower essences (*Star of Bethlehem*, *Rock Rose*, *Impatiens*, *Clematis*, and *Cherry Plum*) intended for use at times of acute mental stress. In the cancer care setting, this would be appropriate for patients or their relatives who are shocked or upset, for example, in relation to bad news about diagnosis, awaiting medical or surgical procedures, dying, or bereavement. However, an individually chosen mixture would work better in some cases.

Some of the remedies are useful mainly for transient emotional imbalances, others for ingrained personality traits. Up to seven remedies may be included in the same mixture but sometimes just one is required.

---

### Case 3

Anne, a young woman suffering from advanced breast cancer, requested a consultation in the hope of finding a natural substitute for sleeping pills. She said the main reason for her insomnia was being unable to relax and 'switch off' from the various projects, professional and social, in which she was still enthusiastically involved despite her frail condition. Although well aware of how ill she was, she described her attitude as extremely positive, saying she was determined to achieve her goals and wanted to 'live as long and good a life as possible'. Ever since her original diagnosis 10 years earlier, she had taken active steps to research information on breast cancer and obtain the best-possible treatments and she had already survived much longer than predicted. Her personality corresponded well with the *Vervain* type and this flower was administered singly. Because of her rapidly progressing disease, and all the other medical treatments she was having, it was difficult to assess the response but she was pleased with the prescription and did sleep better the next few nights. She died peacefully 1 week later.

---

While acute cases often show rapid improvement, others need much more time. With chronic problems, a common pattern of response is the gradual realization of being 'back to my old self again' after a number of weeks. A minority of clients feel a little worse to begin with but then start to improve. Each treatment bottle lasts about 3 weeks and with longer-term cases, it is worth reviewing the selection of flowers before each new mixture is made up. This is because other, deeper aspects of the problem sometimes come to the fore after the presenting outer layers have been dealt with ('peeling the onion').

Many clients seen in the cancer treatment setting will be suffering from transient reactions to acute stress, requiring only brief treatment. Others need to be seen for an extended period, either because their psychological problems are complex and severe or because they are approaching their illness as an opportunity for self-exploration and self-development and find the flowers a valuable aid to this 'transformational response'.

## References

Bach, E. 1933, (revised 1952). *Heal Thyself*. The CW Daniel Company Ltd, Saffron Walden.

Ball, S. 2003, *Teach Yourself Bach Flower Remedies*. Hodder & Stoughton, London.

Chancellor, P. M. 1971, *Illustrated Handbook of the Bach Flower Remedies*. The CW Daniel Company Ltd, Saffron Walden.

Ernst, E. 2002, Flower Remedies: a systematic review of the clinical evidence. *Wien Klin Wochenschr*, vol. **114**, nos. 23–24, pp. 963–6.

Howard, J. 1990, *The Bach Flower Remedies Step by Step*. The CW Daniel Company Ltd, Saffron Walden.

Howard, J. 2007, Do Bach flower remedies have a role to play in pain control? *Complementary therapies in clinical practice*, vol **13**, no. 3, pp. 174–183.

Nelsons, 2006, *Bach Flower Remedies – An Appraisal of the Evidence Base*. PDF document available from enquiries@nelsons.net

Weeks, N. 1940, *The Medical Discoveries of Edward Bach Physician*. The CW Daniel Company Ltd, Saffron Walden.

## Website

www.bachcentre.com

Chapter 12

# Counselling: distress, transitions, and relationships

James Brennan

## Summary

People with cancer, and those close to them, may experience distress relating to many different domains of life as their previous assumptions and expectations are challenged. This descriptive chapter considers how such distress may be acknowledged and assessed, and clients supported through the various transitions imposed by the disease and its treatment, in the context of a therapeutic relationship.

## Introduction

Significant scientific and medical advances over recent years indicate that cancer is often a curable or a chronic condition. Yet, the general public, and most of those diagnosed with cancer, continue to see this disease as a death sentence. A person's view of their future, relationship with others, sense of themselves, and even spiritual beliefs may all be challenged and the consequences are therefore wide-ranging.

It is in the context of this personal turmoil that patients undergo some of medicine's most aggressive interventions. The caricature of surgery, radiotherapy, and chemotherapy as 'slashing, burning, and poisoning' can sometimes be alarmingly near the truth and, for many, surviving cancer remains a formidable test of endurance.

Healthcare policy is increasingly regarding cancer as a chronic illness and recognizing that unprecedented numbers of people are living with the disease and all the distress associated with it. 'Supportive care' encompasses diverse challenges—from pain control, psychological and social care, through to spiritual support. Central to all professional attempts to ameliorate suffering is the therapeutic relationship with the client or patient, most explicitly used in the fields of counselling and psychotherapy.

Healthcare professionals need to communicate all the time in their work and the principles of good communication draw heavily on counselling practice. Formal counselling, by contrast, is a professional relationship in which one person helps the other understand their concerns better and supports them as they adjust to, confront, or tolerate the sources of their distress. This takes place through the medium of language, mostly but not exclusively words. The term 'counselling' is vague, covering a wide range of theories and practices, often leaving practitioners perplexed and confused. Although the limited evidence suggests that it is helpful (Meyer and Mark 1995; Boudioni *et al.* 2000), it is not so in all cases (Moynihan *et al.* 1999) and it not always the most culturally appropriate form of help (Lago and Thompson 1996).

## Acknowledging and assessing distress

All therapeutic relationships begin with a meeting to which both parties bring their own assumptions about the other. The counsellor may have prior information about the client, which influences their perceptions and consequently what they see, hear, and remember. Like all healthcare professionals, counsellors see their patients through the lens of their own life experiences and cultural background, history of loss, and contact with illness.

The client may be making loaded assumptions on the basis of a title such as counsellor, psychologist, or psychotherapist. *Does this mean people think I am not coping? Am I being weak? Do people think I am going mad? What does this say about me?* Any professional title also denotes to the client what is permissible for discussion. *A doctor won't be interested in my sexual difficulties. A counsellor won't be able to help me with my pain.* The first task for the counsellor is to establish a safe, relaxed, and trusting relationship and gently move aside such restraining assumptions.

Many people arrive at their first session either anxious about what they may reveal about themselves or, more often, ready to burst with pent-up emotion. The relief of finally releasing something of the anguish that has been held inside, whether to protect others or to preserve their own dignity, often means that much of the first session may be spent simply hearing the client's distress. The first essential task of the counsellor or any healthcare professional is to acknowledge this. By demonstrating that they are moved by what they have heard, yet are not overwhelmed by it, the counsellor helps to 'contain' the distress. Technically, this is achieved by intense listening, punctuated by occasional reflections and summaries that serve to gather the disparate strands of the client's story into more coherent themes.

People are generally more able to 'read' others from their own culture since they can pick up more easily the subtext and assumptions underlying their spoken words. It may be more challenging for the counsellor to 'get inside' the habitual realities and concerns of people from different cultures, age groups, and lifestyles. Consequently, counsellors must always feel comfortable to clarify *anything* that they do not understand and remain receptive to being corrected.

Clients receiving counselling in the cancer care setting may well be facing active disease, toxic treatments, the possibility of recurrence, or the prospect of death. It is therefore wise to ensure that a brief holistic assessment (covering physical, psychological, social, and spiritual concerns) is made as early as possible and reviewed periodically. Unfortunately, some counsellors without a background in healthcare still see this as unnecessary or compromising.

Counselling is certainly no panacea. Emotional and psychological distress never occurs in isolation; persistent pain, nausea, or fatigue can be as much a source of distress as worries about job security or family finances. Fear is a natural response to uncertainty and depression can be kindled by the loss of hope. Research suggests that the more difficulties or concerns people have, the more their resources become overwhelmed, and the more likely they are to be severely distressed (Cull *et al.* 1995; Parle *et al.* 1996). Yet, rarely do people with cancer express or volunteer their concerns to professionals and rarely are these identified by healthcare staff (Parle *et al.* 1996). It is vital therefore for counsellors not to limit their field of vision but to assess and remain responsive to the broader biological, psychological, social, and spiritual needs of their clients.

A natural place to start the counselling assessment is to explore: (1) the client's most pressing current concerns, (2) the personal and social context, (3) what the client understands about their illness, (4) the implications they see it having on their lives and their relationships, (5) the resources they possess (especially, of course, the support of their family and friends), and (6) their longer-term needs and goals.

This leads naturally to a discussion of the client's personal history, their psychological development and key relationships, thereby providing the *context* for the crisis of their illness. Some sources of distress are past issues which have been brought to life by the changes and threats of the present situation. Those with previous psychological or psychiatric difficulties are especially vulnerable to further problems and may need to be assessed by someone with the appropriate training.

By the end of the initial assessment, the client and counsellor should arrive at clear aims for their work together, even if these subsequently change in the light of developing events. They should also reach an explicit understanding as to the frequency and expected duration of the sessions, as well as other 'boundary issues' such as the limits of confidentiality. Where a more experienced pair of hands is called for, this person should be consulted before any further work is undertaken.

## Transitions

As the client's medical treatment continues, new information about prognosis may emerge. Cancer counselling is therefore provided in 'real time' alongside the unfolding of events over which neither client nor counsellor has much control. A working knowledge of cancer medicine is invaluable here. For the client, uncertainty abounds: *What will the treatment be like? What does this pain mean? Will I be cured and, if not, how long have I got? What will dying be like? What will my test result show? How are my loved ones faring?* Uncertainty can sometimes be decreased by obtaining information but a doctor can seldom tell an individual why *they* got cancer or how long *they* will live.

The counsellor's therapeutic understanding must therefore often develop in the midst of the client's uncertainty and in response to their shifting priorities and changes in focus. In this context, powerful insights can be rendered quickly and part of the counsellor's task may be to temper the rate at which this is happening. Cancer may provide the catalyst for intense individual and interpersonal development but personal growth, even when it is liberating, has to be fashioned from the sometimes unyielding circumstances of life. It is psychologically stressful to have to restructure the knowledge base by which one has lived. It is also deeply sad to be forced to relinquish hopes and aspirations that have been implicitly held for a lifetime. A period of grief, of letting go, must be felt. All this adds to the distress and uncertainty brought about by the illness and its treatment.

For example, as her treatment for breast cancer was coming to an end, a 49-year-old mother of three teenagers was referred with symptoms of depression. She was tearful, irritable, and feeling hopeless. In the first session, she described her disappointment at the lack of support she had had from her family in recent months. As her story unfolded, her rage at the injustice of having supported her husband and children throughout their lives without reciprocation quickly emerged. She spontaneously began to see that she was imprisoned by a system of expectations and assumptions within the family, assumptions that she had helped create and maintain through her own expectations of her role as a mother and wife. With insight came self-blame for having let this situation develop. Her compelling need to subvert this system was thwarted, however, by the emotional and physical exhaustion caused by her diagnosis and treatment, as well as her guilt at the prospect of putting her own needs before others. By helping a client to formulate her own story in this way, counsellors can enable her to make sense of what has happened and re-orientate herself to the often uncertain future that lies ahead.

Most people with cancer need time and space to deal with the shock of suddenly confronting their mortality and having to cope with the uncertainty of this threat. And they are not alone. Partners, family members, and friends may all be contemplating some grim possibilities. This situation may bring unexamined assumptions into sharp relief. *How have I lived my life? What is the true nature of my relationships? How will my loved ones manage if I or they die? What aspirations have I held and now question? What has this illness revealed about me?* These questions are not always consciously articulated but they demand answers nonetheless. 'Unfinished business', such as guilt about a past relationship, becomes active and urgent again although, at the same time, it can feel dangerous and presumptuous to make any plans for the future. Existing in the present, 'from day to day', is often the more comfortable option.

The task of the counsellor is to support the client through this storm of uncertainty by helping them marshal their own strengths and resources as they make sense of what they have been through and the challenges that lie ahead. If counsellors are familiar with some of the common themes that people with cancer have to grapple with, and the processes of adjustment they go through, they can be more receptive and responsive to their needs.

Many of these core life assumptions have been formally summarized in the *Social-Cognitive Transition Model of Adjustment* (Brennan 2001). This simple model emphasizes that throughout our lives, we develop assumptions and expectations about the world, drawn from our social and cultural environments. These assumptions include unspoken beliefs about ourselves and other people. In turn, what we learn about life alters these assumptions and expectations. Much of what we learn is 'implicit knowledge' (in technical terms 'preconscious') or embodied (skills, habits, etc.) and these mental maps of the world enable each unfolding moment to be experienced as part of a more or less continuous and coherent whole.

When our most deep-seated assumptions fail to adequately make sense of a new situation, we are left disorientated, afraid, and potentially traumatized. The unreal, dreamlike state of shock following a diagnosis of cancer is a powerful example. Besides the psychological adjustment required, patients may experience challenges in employment and domestic arrangements, social conditions, relationships with other people, and spiritual beliefs, at the same time as undergoing harsh treatments.

Alongside the need to integrate these new realities into their lives, people with cancer are naturally *resistant* to changing their previously coherent understanding of the world, especially if it requires a major reorganization of their mental maps. Yet, this is what adjustment to cancer often entails. Denial and avoidance are therefore entirely normal psychological defence mechanisms that serve to maintain a level of continuity and coherence against the threat of fragmentation (Mollon 2002). They enable new information to be absorbed more gradually, thereby reducing distress. Denial only becomes a 'problem' when people refuse to accept the treatment that is being offered or are unable to communicate openly with their loved ones.

Both the individual and those close to them are in transition, in the sense that their core assumptions about the world have been violated or discredited, and with time they will feel compelled to adjust them. These core assumptions are summarized below under five headings. These are very loose categories— there are of course endless ways of carving up human experience. All of the following can be fertile ground for the development of emotional distress as well as, sometimes, personal growth (Brennan 2004).

## Life trajectory

All our lives are structured around often implicit and unspoken plans, goals, and assumptions about the future. Cancer has been described as an 'amputation of the future' (Frank-Stromberg et al. 1984) in which these assumptions are fractured, if not permanently shattered. Re-examining one's aspirations can be helpful if it leads to new priorities and more meaningful goals, but often it leads to a painful grieving process during which long-held dreams and ambitions are gradually relinquished.

After a few encounters with 'bad news', people often feel they would be tempting fate to make any firm plans, while prolonged pain, nausea, or fatigue may remove the will to make them anyway. However, without things to achieve and look forward to, we are in danger of losing hope, meaning, and self-confidence. For people facing the certainty of their death, adjustment may entail an enquiry into the value and meaning of their lives and how best to spend their remaining time.

David Spiegel has pointed to the value of 'detoxifying death' by enabling clients to talk about their fears (Spiegel and Diamond 2001), which is often difficult to do in other relationships. The cancer counsellor must create safety if people wish to examine their deepest fears. By helping clients to integrate their illness with their past experiences, counsellors can enable them to re-engage productively with their present and future lives, however long or short these may be.

## Attachments

John Bowlby (1988) described how, as we grow up, we develop deeply held assumptions concerning the nature of our relationships and how these will meet our dependency needs. When threatened or in a state of dangerous ambiguity, our instinct is to *attach* ourselves to the secure base of a trusted parental figure. As we grow into adulthood, this need for a secure base gradually becomes projected onto others, such as partners, and authority figures, such as doctors.

Whatever its objective prognosis, cancer confronts people with the threat of permanent separation from loved ones and the very nature of these attachments becomes suddenly clear. The threat posed by the disease can reawaken childhood attachment needs as people unconsciously search for a parental figure. Patients understandably look to their doctors for this kind of care and authority but they also turn to their loved ones for emotional and practical support. The reality that follows, however, sometimes violates assumptions about relationships that may have developed over many years. Among couples, it can lead to resentful adversity at a time when both parties often need each other more than ever; therefore, when counselling couples, it is imperative to attend to the attachment assumptions of both partners.

Parents must contemplate the possibility that they will not watch their children grow up, couples must work through their disappointed expectations of one another as one of them learns to be a patient and the other a caring support, and single people must face the challenge of making new friends and dating, such as when to talk about their cancer and its treatment, how much to tell, and bearing rejection if this occurs (Brennan 2004). Families must undergo role changes while still attending to the developmental needs of all their members. These are not trivial challenges but demand open, honest communication among people who may lack a history of openness with one another. Men and women do not always share the same language of care or the capacity to communicate feelings and there are often different cultural expectations regarding what should be expressed to whom.

The counsellor can help clients reconsider their assumptions about their key attachments and support the client if he or she chooses to challenge them. Counsellors can offer support and 'rehearsal time' if clients need to reveal painful information about their prognosis to loved ones, such as children. In addition, they can help clients reflect on and resolve previously difficult relationships. The client–counsellor relationship itself offers a useful medium through which to understand the client's internal working models about their key relationships.

## Control and Self-worth

The third area of the assumptive world that is undermined by cancer is the client's sense of self-worth and personal control. A belief in personal control is integral to a person's self-concept and self-esteem, as well as the maintenance of non-depressed mood (Taylor and Brown 1988) and the counsellor has an important role in helping clients restore their sense of value and control. Long courses of treatment tend to disengage clients from many of the occupational, family, and social roles that formerly provided regular feedback about their value and power in society, leading them to doubt their skills, talents, and personal qualities. Cancer is also frequently seen as an uncontrollable threat and this can induce a sense of helplessness and a dependence on others, particularly medical staff, to make the situation safe again. This loss of control is compounded by having to adopt the powerless role of a patient within the complex and intimidating world of cancer medicine.

In addition to these treatment-related assaults on the client's sense of their worth and power may come the reactivation of unresolved issues from the past. Current events may resonate with earlier traumas involving loss, separation, or abuse that then require therapeutic attention. In one case, a woman was unconsciously reminded of her repressed childhood sexual abuse as she lay under a radiotherapy machine. Over the next few days, she experienced intrusive momentary flashbacks, which in the context of counselling she was able to piece together and subsequently work through (Brennan 2000). Counsellors can also do much to restore clients' self-worth and control by helping them to 'encapsulate' the illness within one part of their lives, rather than allowing it to dominate or define them.

## The body

Our bodies are so central to our identity or self-concept that we rarely consider the assumptions we have developed about them. However, it is through the sensory apparatus and functions of the body that we interact with the world and one another. The effects of disfiguring treatment, noxious symptoms, and chronic disability can undermine life-long assumptions about the reliability, image, capabilities, and sensation of the body, as well as its social capital. Chemotherapy, radiotherapy, and hormone treatment can have direct effects on mood, while symptoms such as pain and fatigue can wear down the client's resilience, leaving them emotionally as well as physically exhausted. The particular site of the cancer or the side effects of the treatment may hold particular meaning for the client beyond their more obvious implications.

Following treatment, many patients retain a residual suspicion, if not a morbid fear, that one day the body will once again provide shelter for the enemy. For a smaller number, this takes the form of intrusive ruminations or compulsive urges to check for signs that the disease has returned

(Somerfield *et al.* 1999). Living with uncertainty is therefore often a major focus for supportive counselling.

## Existential–Spiritual

Being able to contemplate one's mortality is often considered a defining feature of what it is to be human. The spiritual side of a person is that which expresses a person's deepest convictions about the nature of existence. Questions of existential meaning usually involve notions of fundamental causation and purpose and the preciousness of being alive. These questions are naturally important to people, especially so when in mortal danger, because it is human nature to struggle to understand the world we inhabit and to anticipate our future.

The search for meaning and purpose is not limited to the spiritual beliefs embodied in formal religions. Everyone has core beliefs about the nature of existence and these are not always framed with reference to a god. Following cancer, people often appear to be more concerned with constructing a moral summary or overview of their existence in the world, of asking the questions '*Why me?*' or '*What is the point of going on if I will eventually die from this disease?*' The wish to attribute blame or causation to something or someone is common and understandable. God may be an obvious target for blame, although the need for accountability can become displaced onto others such as doctors or employers or the self ('I should have stopped smoking').

Such existential–spiritual questions can leave people highly distressed, lost in a sea without reference points. Counsellors have no better answers to these questions than anyone else but they should not shy away from them because many clients lack the structure and support provided by a formal religious affiliation or any other context in which to explore them. Counselling can help restore existential meaning through a clarification of core spiritual beliefs and ethics. Conducting a life review involves the client telling the story of their lives so that 'unfinished business' from the past (regrets, conflicts, anger, missed opportunities, etc.) can be better understood and integrated into a more coherent life narrative. For those with limited time, counselling can help clients find a way to 'live life to the full' or develop a mindful awareness of unfolding experience or, indeed, to face death with a sense of completion.

These five domains are not exhaustive but they provide a framework for understanding some of the emotional concerns that people with cancer commonly need to address. The aim of cancer counselling should be to help clients absorb the implications of their illness so that by recognizing the core assumptions that have been violated, they can equip themselves with a more effective mental model for the future. The focus is on helping people in crisis regain their sense of orientation, take charge of their lives, find peace in their emotions, and sometimes restore a sense of meaning. It is about supporting people as they re-engage productively and creatively with their ever-changing lives. Reviving a person's spirit often means helping them find new hope through creativity and goals that offer achievement and pleasure, although admittedly this can sometimes be a huge challenge during advanced disease, when what has been relinquished must be grieved.

## Therapeutic relationships

The most powerful active ingredient in counselling is the client–counsellor relationship. Unlike other social relationships, the support provided in counselling has clear and explicit boundaries. The special skills of the counsellor are not about possessing expert knowledge but creating conditions for the client such that they become clearer about their values, resources, and capacity for self-determination. In the context of cancer, the client may not be able to speak openly to their normal sources of social support—their families, partners, and friends. These people are not only having to manage their own fears and distress but may be unhelpfully insisting that the client adopt a resolutely 'positive' stance. In contrast, the safe containment of the counselling relationship should enable clients to venture further and explore the fears and losses that are distressing them.

Finding words to explore the meaning of recent events enables people to integrate these events with their core assumptions about the world, and prevents difficult experiences from becoming dissociated or being split off. Furthermore, talking through a fear of the future equips one with the means to manage it. The very act of trying to put diffuse thoughts and feelings into words gives them shape and form that often makes events appear more controllable, predictable, and therefore more manageable. It helps people consider the problems they face and the options and resources available to them and it provides reassurance when making decisions. Much psychological therapy relies upon this process but it is only achieved if the client–counsellor relationship facilitates it. Carl Rogers (1961) emphasized that the counsellor should demonstrate *empathy* (constantly working towards a better understanding of what it must feel like to be the client and being able to convey this understanding back to them), *unconditional positive regard* (a stance of care and respect regardless of what the client says, unconditionally in the way that a parent cares for their child, attempting to understand and value the client rather than judge them), and *authenticity* (being genuine with the client, not acting the part of a professional but being honest, open, and natural in one's responses). More than any other, this quality of genuineness is essential in cancer counselling. Research has confirmed that people with cancer value psychotherapists who are seen to be genuinely caring human beings (MacCormack *et al.* 2001). This need for here-and-now authentic human contact may, in time, lead to more relaxed boundaries concerning personal disclosures by the counsellor, *provided* that it is always in the service of the relationship, it is in the client's best interests, and both the counsellor and client feel comfortable with the content.

In short, the client needs to experience the counsellor as being entirely *present* in the room, not concerned about other things but wholly ready to *hear* the client. And, finally, when the client may feel it is a struggle to survive in the face of overwhelming change and uncertainty, he or she must feel that they are meeting someone who is genuinely 'on their side'.

People have powerful attachment needs in times of uncertainty and danger, and doctors, counsellors, and other healthcare professionals represent figures of authority in whom clients are keen to invest their trust. Similarly, the emotional bond between spouses or partners is often derived from childhood needs and is based on the assumption that one or both of them will provide protection and care to the other when required ('in sickness and in health'). Of course, all clients have their unique history of attachments so, whenever possible, counsellors should take time to consider the attachment style of their client by exploring their relationship history. This may inform the relationship that the client and counsellor subsequently create.

Depending on childhood experiences, attachment styles vary enormously. People with a secure attachment history believe that they are worthy of care and that others can be trusted to provide this; consequently, they are more likely to seek out effective support (Schmidt *et al.* 2002). In contrast, insecure patterns of attachments can range from the avoidance of intimacy at one end of the continuum to a clinging dependence at the other. For example, the loss of a parent early in life may lead to insecure attachments later on, with undue dependency, separation anxiety, and anticipation of further losses. These attachment styles will often be borne out in the relationship the client builds with their current caregivers, other family members, and healthcare staff. Moreover, their attachment needs will find expression in the relationship they form with their counsellor and, conversely, will be affected by it. The feelings that emerge between a client and a counsellor are known as the *transference*.

## Transference

On the basis of their previous experience of other relationships, clients project their feelings and assumptions onto the counsellor, other healthcare professionals, and sometimes whole teams. The counsellor may be unconsciously seen as similar to a key figure in the client's life; in other words, the client may expect the relationship with the counsellor to follow a habitual pattern. If counsellors are able to observe how the client relates to them (the transference), they may gain valuable insights into the clients' attachment style and their other relationships. It is, therefore, important for counsellors to consider who or what they may unconsciously represent for the client and vice versa.

For example, a client who has been abused or neglected as a child may have a dismissing or testing attitude towards the counsellor until they can feel safe to trust them. In contrast, someone who is perceived as 'stuck' on a ward may be demanding constant reassurances from the healthcare team and, due to a fear of abandonment, be reluctant to leave their care. Other people may defend against their own dependency needs by appearing to be resolutely autonomous. Men have often been raised to equate autonomy with maturity and may therefore feel uncomfortable about being dependent on others. In their search for certainty, clients often view counsellors as parental figures and may subtly and unconsciously seek reassurance from them about their illness and its future course. Counsellors can feel pressurized to collude with an overly positive interpretation of events. Yet, their job is to contain and acknowledge the client's feelings, not to provide empty reassurances.

Moreover, what of the counsellor's feelings? Counsellors too have attachment histories, and cultural assumptions, and these must be carefully examined to illuminate whether feelings in the consulting room are emanating from the client or from the counsellor's *counter-transference* (feelings towards the client). The client's age, gender, or individual vulnerability may resonate with the counsellor's memory of earlier relationships, which he/she may feel driven to undo or recreate. Similarly, the client's concerns may awaken unresolved distress in the counsellor, who either avoids these issues or over-identifies with them. The relationship between counsellor and client is reciprocal and both sides of the transference relationship should be considered. Possibly the most sophisticated yet valuable source of information available to the counsellor is his or her changing feelings towards the client. It takes considerable practice to capture these feelings at the moment one is having them, yet they can provide powerful insights into the client's unexpressed concerns.

If a safe and trusting relationship can be established, clients will perceive their consultations as a time entirely for themselves, a place to confront the unthinkable or unspeakable, and a space to consider their assumptions and worries. Once the dread of putting these thoughts into words has been overcome, many concerns evaporate or can be shelved. People who have talked through their fears about dying and the fate of their loved ones may feel reassured by having imagined more realistically what may be entailed. Consequently, they are less likely to suffer with intrusive ruminations and their distress diminishes as a result. Finally, cancer counselling is not always as gloomy as this chapter may suggest. Clients often have hilarious stories related to their illness experience, which they are keen to share. Humour and creativity are reminders that there are many qualities and facets of the individual that are not affected by cancer.

In the context of a life-threatening disease, the end of counselling sessions can be particularly challenging; yet, if handled well, this stage of the work may be especially therapeutic. The ending has a powerful parallel with what happens to all relationships, especially at the end of life. It provides an opportunity to reflect on what has been valuable, acknowledge feelings of loss, and consider the future. It is important that the counsellor does not shy away from discussing the ending, but rather provides a model of someone who is able to confront and manage the difficult feelings it evokes.

## Conclusion

Counsellors characteristically work with the biographical and interpersonal aspects of people's lives, rather than the physical, social, or spiritual. However, cancer is an uncertain and unpredictable disease with wide-ranging implications. Cancer counsellors therefore have an ethical duty to be sufficiently aware of these other concerns to be able to refer patients on to relevant specialists when their own level of competence or knowledge is breached. Certainly, where psychological distress is long-standing or particularly complex, an early referral to, or close supervision from, a mental health specialist such as a clinical psychologist or psychiatrist should be arranged.

It can be a rare privilege but always a huge responsibility to share the private, emotional, and spiritual life of a person by virtue of their trust. The job satisfaction of working with clients who, confronted by their mortality, find the courage to transform their lives can be compelling. However, it can be spiritually draining to enter the inner world of other people and try to support them as they face the possibility or prospect of their life ending. It can be arresting to consider the apparently arbitrary way that cancer chooses its victims and to be reminded of one's own mortality. Counsellors must learn to tolerate the sometimes powerful feelings of helplessness as they bear witness to their clients' anguish and distress at an extraordinarily vulnerable time in their lives. In short, cancer counselling should not be undertaken lightly or provided by someone insufficiently trained, supported, or supervised.

All cancer counsellors should have regular access to clinical supervision and support, in which they can monitor and regulate their stress levels by discussing their feelings and reactions towards their clients. They should strive to recognize blind spots and areas of difficulty or avoidance, identify unexamined assumptions brought to their work, and discuss ethical doubts or strong feelings about particular clients. Finally, counsellors should consider the balance and boundaries between their professional and personal lives, so as to safeguard their own personal and existential development.

## References

Boudioni, M., Mossman, J., Boulton, M., Ramirez, A., Moynihan, C. & Leydon, G. 2000, An evaluation of a cancer counselling service, *European Journal of Cancer Care*, vol. 9, pp. 212–20.

Bowlby, J. 1988, *A Secure Base – Clinical Applications of Attachment Theory*. London: Routledge.

Brennan, J. 2000, Changing tack: the importance of the therapeutic relationship, *Primary Care and Cancer*, vol. 20, pp. 31–4.

Brennan, J. 2001, Adjustment to cancer - coping or personal transition?, *Psycho-Oncology*, vol. 10, pp. 1–18.

Brennan, J. 2004, *Cancer in Context: A Practical Guide to Supportive Care*. Oxford University Press, Oxford.

Cull, A., Stewart, M. & Altman, D. G. 1995, Assessment of and intervention for psychosocial problems in routine oncology practice, *British Journal of Cancer*, vol. 72, pp. 229–35.

Frank-Stromberg, M., Wright, P. S., Segalla, M. & Diekmann, J. 1984, Psychological impact of the 'cancer' diagnosis, *Oncology Nursing Forum*, vol. 11, pp. 16–22.

Lago, C. & Thompson, J. 1996, *Race, Culture and Counselling*. Open University Press, Buckingham.

MacCormack, T., Simonian, J., Lim, J. *et al.* 2001, Someone who cares: A qualitative investigation of cancer patients' experience of psychotherapy. *Psycho-Oncology*, vol. 10, pp. 52–65.

Meyer, T. J. & Mark, M. M. 1995, Effects of psychosocial interventions with adult cancer patients: a meta-analysis of randomized experiments, *Health Psychology*, vol. 14, pp. 101–08.

Mollon, P. 2002, *Releasing the Self: The Healing Legacy of Heinz Kohut*. Wiley, Chichester.

Moynihan, C., Horwich, A. & Bliss, J. 1999, Counselling is not appropriate for all patients with cancer, *British Medical Journal*, vol. 318, p. 128.

Parle, M., Jones, B. & Maguire, P. 1996, Maladaptive coping and affective disorders among cancer patients, *Psychological Medicine*, vol. 26, pp. 735–44.

Rogers, C. R. 1961, *On Becoming a Person*. Houghton Mifflin: Boston, MA.

Schmidt, S., Nachtigall, C., Wuethrich-Martone, O. & Strauss, B. 2002, Attachment and coping with chronic disease, *Journal of Psychosomatic Research*, vol. 53, 763–73.

Somerfield, M. R., Stefanek, M. E., Smith, T. J. & Padberg, J. J. 1999, A systems model for adaptation to somatic distress among cancer survivors, *Psycho-Oncology*, vol. 8, pp. 334–43.

Spiegel, D. & Diamond, S. 2001, Psychosocial interventions in cancer – group therapy techniques. In (eds) Baum, A. & Anderson, B. L. *Psychosocial Interventions in Cancer*. American Psychological Association, Washington.

Taylor, S. E. & Brown, J. D. 1988, Illusion and well-being: a social psychological perspective on mental health, *Psychological Bulletin*, vol. 103, pp. 193–210.

## Chapter 13

# Exercise

Margaret L McNeely and Kerry S Courneya

## Summary

Increasing attention has been directed towards survivorship issues for individuals diagnosed with cancer. Preliminary research has shown that appropriately prescribed exercise training programs are associated with low complication rates and numerous beneficial effects. On the basis of current evidence, the American Cancer Society recommends that cancer survivors participate in regular physical activity (Brown *et al.* 2003). This chapter provides an overview of exercise as an intervention in the rehabilitation of patients with cancer and cancer survivors and includes recommendations for exercise programming based on research evidence and the clinical experience of the authors.

## Definitions and benefits of physical activity and exercise

Physical activity is defined as any bodily movement requiring the contraction of skeletal muscles that results in a substantial increase in energy expenditure over resting levels (Bouchard 1994; ACSM 2006). This may include leisure-time physical activity and/or occupational and household physical activity. Exercise is defined as a form of leisure-time physical activity that is planned, structured, and usually performed on a repeated basis over an extended period of time. Exercise is prescribed specifically with the intent of improving fitness, performance, and/or health. Current public health guidelines recommend daily physical activity and/or formal exercise at a level that is equivalent to 30 minute of brisk walking, five or more days per week.

The benefits of regular physical activity and exercise can be viewed as a combination of psychosocial and physiological effects. More specifically, the physiological effects of cardiorespiratory, or aerobic, exercise training include significant changes in both cardiovascular and pulmonary systems (McArdle *et al.* 2001). This results in an improved ability of the cardiorespiratory system to take in, extract, deliver, and use oxygen and to remove waste products from the body tissues. Regular exercise also reduces resting and submaximal heart rate, systolic and diastolic blood pressure, and can alter body composition by decreasing body fat (Hall and Brody 1999).

The physiological effects of progressive resistance exercise (PRE), or strength, training include positive changes in musculoskeletal fitness and improvements in the tensile strength of tendons and ligaments. PRE can be used to maintain or improve bone density (Hall and Brody 1999). PRE training programs have also succeeded in improving several indicators of health status, for example, blood pressure, heart rate, glucose metabolism, obesity, and functional status (Hall and Brody 1999).

Regular exercise can also aid and enhance psychological well-being by improving mood and reducing anxiety. Moreover, exercise has the potential to lower mortality rates by decreasing the risk of cardiovascular diseases, cancers, and the development of Type 2 diabetes (ACSM, 2006). Finally, participation in regular excercise appears to lower the risk of developing depression, and improves symptoms of depression in individuals with the condition (ACSM, 2006).

## Overview of research on physical activity and exercise in the cancer population

Several studies have examined physical activity and exercise behaviour in cancer populations. Cancer treatment has been found to have a significantly negative effect on exercise participation that is not completely recovered post-treatment (Jones et al. 2004). The percentage of cancer survivors who exercise regularly is as low as 16–20% (Jones and Courneya 2002).

Recently, observational data from the Nurse's Health Study showed a protective association between increased physical activity following breast cancer diagnosis and recurrence, cancer-related mortality, and overall mortality (Holmes et al. 2005). This protective effect was shown for physical activity levels that met or exceeded the equivalent of four to five 30-min sessions of brisk walking per week. Similar findings were reported in two observational studies examining physical activity and colorectal cancer (Meyerhardt et al. 2006a,b). These research findings suggest a need for, and potential benefit from, interventions to promote physical activity and exercise across cancer-related time periods.

### Intervention trials

Exercise may provide an effective means of preventing deconditioning and improving physical functioning, both during and following cancer treatment.

Three recent meta-analyses (Stevinson *et al.* 2004; Schmitz *et al.* 2005; McNeely *et al.* 2006) have all concluded that there is evidence to support exercise as an intervention for patients with cancer and cancer survivors. Although this evidence has been the result of trials primarily performed with patients with early-stage breast cancer, given the low complication rates and numerous beneficial effects (Table 13.1), the evidence is viewed as sufficient to support exercise as a rehabilitation intervention with other types of cancer.

## Treatment-related side effects

In this section, we focus on common side effects from cancer treatment that may require consideration prior to exercise testing and programming.

*Fatigue* is the most prevalent side effect of cancer treatment, occurring in 60–90% of survivors (Portenoy and Itri 1999). Fatigue may be described as a lack of energy and tiredness that interferes with day-to-day functioning. Exercise tolerance may be difficult to determine as the individual suffering from fatigue may be unable to exercise for more than a few minutes before becoming too tired to continue. In these cases, exercise testing and training may be best carried out on special equipment such as a low-wattage cycle ergometer to accommodate lower levels of strength and fitness. Interval training, where rest periods of 30 seconds to 1 minute are interspersed with 2- to 3-min bouts of exercise, may be more manageable as a starting point.

**Table 13.1** Possible benefits of exercise during and following cancer treatment

**Psychological**

- Quality of life
- Vigour
- Mood
- Self-report of physical functioning
- Fatigue

**Physiological**

- Objective physical functioning and cardiorespiratory fitness
- Physiological outcomes: e.g., haemoglobin, hospital stay
- Symptoms during treatment: e.g., pain, disability, infection
- Body composition

*Pain* is another prevalent symptom, occurring in up to 50% of patients with cancer (Yeager *et al.* 2000). Whether exercise is appropriate as an intervention depends on the source of the pain. An increase in pain either during or following exercise is a sign of doing too much and in the early recovery period following surgery or radiation therapy (RT), too much exercise may inhibit the healing process. Exercise may be prescribed to address deficits as a result of cancer treatment (e.g. shoulder restriction following mastectomy) and is usually directed at restoring motion, strength, and function within the limits of the pain. For chronic pain syndromes, the focus of an exercise program may be to return to the highest level of overall function in conjunction with a pain management program.

*Peripheral neuropathy* is a common result of chemotherapy-induced inflammation, injury, or degeneration of the peripheral nerve fibres (Armstrong *et al.* 2005). Early symptoms of peripheral neuropathy include tingling, numbness, and burning in the fingers and toes. These symptoms can persist for months to years following treatment and may progress to pain, loss of deep tendon reflexes, reduced muscle tone, and sensory changes. Loss of sensation in the upper extremities may make gripping of equipment problematic and unsafe. For example, free weights with hand straps may be preferred over standard dumbbell weights. Loss of sensation in the lower extremities may increase the risk of falls and injury if the individual cannot sense the position of his/her limbs while walking. In these cases, use of a recumbent cycle ergometer may be a preferred mode of exercise over treadmill walking.

*The integrity of muscle and bone* can be affected by cancer and its treatments. For example, steroid-induced myopathy commonly occurs in patients taking high doses of fluorinated corticosteroids and is characterized by weakness in the proximal muscles of the limbs and neck flexors (Batchelor *et al.* 1997). Resistance exercises that target postural muscles as well as these vulnerable muscle groups may serve to attenuate declines in muscular strength. Chemotherapy, alone or in combination with RT, can also lead to osteopenia. The effects of RT on bone include functional limitations, osteonecrosis, osteoporosis, increased susceptibility to fractures, and poor healing (Moore 2000). In these cases, integrity of the bone is the primary concern. Carefully prescribed PRE and/or weight-bearing exercises such as walking, stepping, and stair climbing may be beneficial as an adjunct to pharmacological interventions, provided the risk of fracture and falls is low.

*Cardiac complications* may occur with chemotherapeutic agents, hormone therapy, and immunotherapy (Floyd 2005). Presentations range from relatively benign arrhythmias to potentially serious conditions such as cardiomyopathy. Medical supervision of exercise testing is essential for those who have undergone chemotherapy with potentially cardiotoxic agents. Close supervision of the cancer survivor during exercise sessions is recommended to ensure an appropriate cardiovascular response to exercise.

*Changes in weight and body composition* occur with cancer and its treatments and may reduce health-related quality of life, increase the risk of other disease conditions, and reduce overall survival. For example, treatment-related weight gain is common in both breast and prostate cancer and results in increased visceral fat mass and loss of lean muscle mass (Goodwin 1999). In contrast, weight loss affects approximately 50% of all cancer survivors (Ardies 2002). Cancer cachexia, or severe weight loss due to cancer and/or its treatments, is known to negatively affect skeletal muscle metabolism, leading to muscle wasting and weakness (Ardies 2002). In cases where weight and body composition are the focus, a multidisciplinary approach that considers both nutritional issues and overall energy expenditure is required.

## Exercise programming

Medical evaluation of the cancer survivor is recommended prior to participation in an exercise program. The medical evaluation must include screening of risk factors for and identification of any symptoms related to cardiovascular, pulmonary, and metabolic diseases and any comorbid conditions that may preclude exercise participation. Information must be collected on important diagnostic and treatment variables associated with cancer, such as the type and stage of disease and type of cancer treatment. Any acute or chronic impairment related to cancer and/or cancer treatment must also be identified (Courneya *et al.* 2004).

The results of the medical evaluation provide the exercise professional with information to guide exercise testing and prescription. A measure of exercise tolerance should be performed prior to commencement of the exercise programme. Cardiorespiratory exercise tolerance may be quantified through maximal exercise testing (e.g. peak oxygen consumption) or predicted from a submaximal exercise test or a test of functional capacity such as the 6-min walk test (McArdle *et al.* 2001). Musculoskeletal exercise tolerance may be determined by muscular strength testing using the one-repetition maximum (1-RM) test. Maximal strength testing may not be appropriate for elderly or impaired patients with cancer and in these cases, the 1-RM may be estimated by a submaximal test, such as the 10-RM test, or tested isometrically using hand-held dynamometry or cable tensiometry (McArdle 2001). We recommend medical supervision of exercise testing of patients with cancer and cancer survivors as per recommended guidelines for other chronic diseases.

## Exercise prescription

The optimal exercise prescription in terms of dose–response relationship is currently not known (Courneya *et al.* 2004). Furthermore, as the response to exercise may not be linear or predictable during adjuvant cancer treatment, we propose exercise prescription options for the post-cancer treatment phase. A structured exercise program includes a warm up, the exercise phase, and a cool-down phase (ACSM 2006). The exercise program should include components such as cardiorespiratory fitness, muscular strength and endurance, and flexibility training. A summary of exercise prescription options for the post-cancer treatment rehabilitation phase is provided in Table 13.2.

## Cardiorespiratory exercise training

The cardiorespiratory or aerobic component of the exercise session involves activities such as walking, swimming, and cycling. Although walking may be the preferred mode of exercise, numerous alternatives exist for aerobic training

**Table 13.2** Exercise prescription options

| Type of physical activity | Prescription factors for the post-treatment rehabilitation phase | Suggested measurement methods/ tools to guide exercise | Comments |
|---|---|---|---|
| Low intensity endurance exercises/activities | Exercises or exercise programs that are performed at a threshold below that required to improve cardiorespiratory fitness (e.g., regular walking rather than brisk walking) Frequency: most if not all days of the week | Heart rate monitor or measurement of pulse Perceived exertion using Borg scale: rating of 10–12 'fairly light' on the Borg 6–20 scale | May also include formal exercise programs such as Tai Chi Chuan, Yoga, dance/ movement therapy |
| Exercise to improve cardiorespiratory fitness | Moderate intensity exercise (e.g., 40–60% HRR[1]) 20–45 minutes, 3–5 days per week | Heart rate monitor/pulse oximeter and blood pressure Perceived exertion using Borg scale: rating of 12–15 'somewhat hard' on the Borg 6–20 scale | Threshold level of intensity: 40–50% HRR to yield improvements in cardiorespiratory fitness |

**Table 13.2** (cont.)

| Type of physical activity | Prescription factors for the post treatment rehabilitation phase | Suggested measurement methods/ tools to guide exercise | Comments |
|---|---|---|---|
| Exercise to improve muscular strength and endurance | 8–10 exercises of major muscle groups of upper and lower extremities and trunk Start with lowest weight on rack or alternatively at 30% of 1 RM$^2$ progressing to 60–70% of 1 RM over a 12-week period 10–15 repetitions, 1–3 sets, 2–3 days per week | Heart rate monitor Perceived exertion using Borg scale: rating of 13 'somewhat hard' to 15 'hard' on the Borg 6–20 scale | Monitor symptoms of pain and fatigue, delayed muscle soreness; reduce/ adjust workload if worsening of symptoms with exercise is observed |
| Exercise to improve flexibility | 2–4 stretches of each muscle group Each stretch held for 10–30 seconds, frequency: 2–3 days per week | Goniometer to measure joint range/Sit and reach test | Alternate activities include Yoga and dance/movement therapy |

[1]HRR, heart rate reserve
[2]RM, repetition maximum

such as use of an arm ergometer and elliptical cross trainer or participation in low-impact aerobic dance class. The goal, in the initial phases of the exercise program, is to first reach target frequency (e.g. 3–5 days per week), then duration (at least 20 minutes, which can be broken into shorter bouts of 5–10 minutes), and finally progress to the desired intensity (e.g. 40–60% of heart rate reserve). The intensity of the exercise should begin at the low end of the desired range (e.g. 40% of heart rate reserve) and progress slowly into the heart rate range as adaptation occurs. This gradual progression of exercise will allow for musculoskeletal adaptation and help avoid injury.

## Resistance exercise training

The resistance training component of the program should last 20–30 minutes and, if possible, should follow the aerobic component. We recommend a therapeutic approach to resistance exercise training that starts either by using the 'lightest weight on the rack' or, if 1-RM data is available, by using a low-resistance weight (e.g. approximately 30% of 1 RM). The individual performs 8–10 repetitions and is gradually progressed to 12–15 repetitions. Initially, the individual should be closely monitored to ensure that exercises are performed correctly. The resistance level is increased once the individual can complete two sets of 12–15 repetitions with good technique and posture. Heart rate and perceived exertion can be used to monitor intensity during the resistance exercise session. The heart rate should not exceed the maximum intensity for the aerobic exercise component. From a more practical standpoint, fatigue should occur by, but not earlier than, the last two to three repetitions of the second set of a given exercise. Resistance training should be performed two to three times per week, with a minimum of 48 hours between training sessions (Table 13.2).

The response to aerobic and resistance exercise, in terms of post-exercise fatigue and muscular soreness, should be evaluated following each exercise session. Any secondary muscular soreness should resolve within 48 hours. Excessive fatigue and/or muscular soreness following an exercise session are suggestive of overtraining and require a reduction in the training volume (e.g. lower intensity and/or shorter duration, lower resistance level, and/or fewer repetitions).

## Flexibility training

A flexibility training program should include a regular set of stretching and range of motion exercises intended to lengthen shortened muscles and/or increase joint range of motion. Ideally, flexibility exercises should focus on large and/or two-joint muscles (e.g. pectorals, quadriceps, hamstrings, gastrocnemius) (Hall and Brody 1999). The choice of range of motion and flexibility exercises can be individualized, for example, to address adaptive shortening of muscles or connective tissue as a result of surgery and/or RT. Flexibility exercises should always consist of slow, static stretches held for 10–30 seconds. During stretching, relaxed breathing should be encouraged. Further details on prescription factors are provided in Table 13.2.

## Special considerations

It is important to note that health benefits may be realized by simply increasing daily physical activity (e.g. 30 minutes of accumulated activity per day). For the less active and/or more deconditioned survivor, the prescription may start by simply encouraging a more active lifestyle (e.g. take the stairs, walk instead of driving), with the goal of increasing daily physical activity to levels advocated by public health guidelines. This lower intensity exercise can be incorporated into the individual's lifestyle (Table 13.2). As activity levels improve, the individual may be more willing and able to incorporate a formal exercise component into day-to-day life.

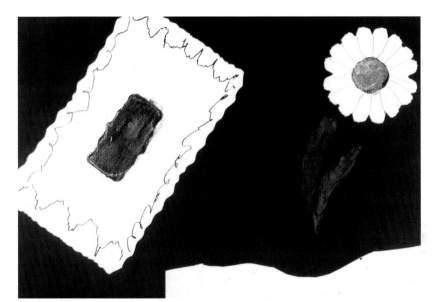

**Colour Plate 1** *'Hope.'*

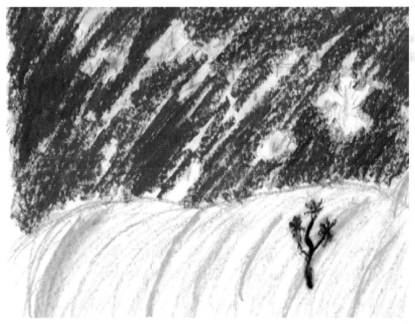

**Colour Plate 2** *'Star-flower.'*

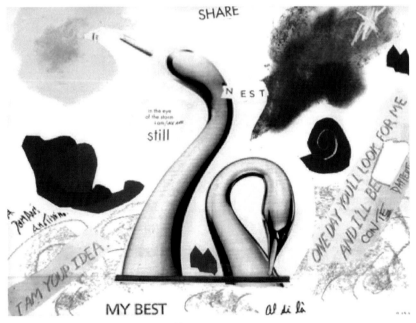

**Colour Plate 3** *'Beyond the beyond.'*

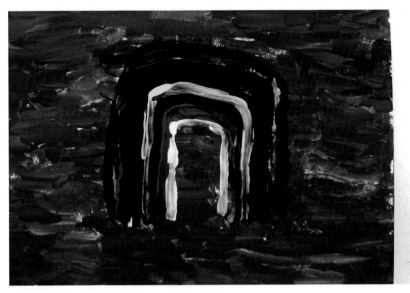

**Colour Plate 4** *'The bridge towards the unknown.'*

## A MODEL OF INTEGRATIVE MEDICAL MUSIC PSYCHOTHERAPY

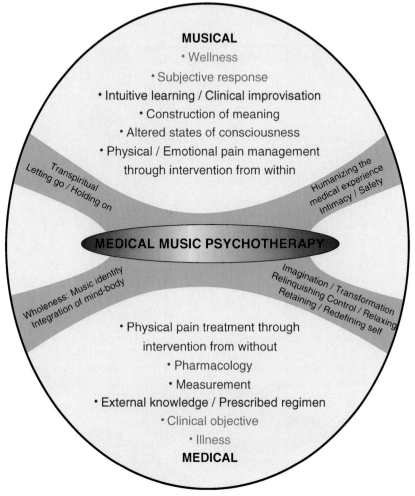

**Colour Plate 5**

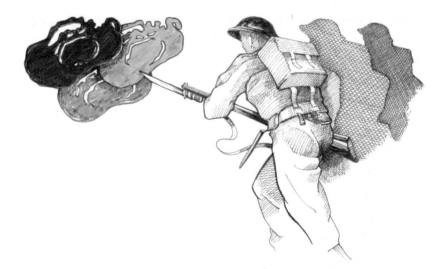

**Colour Plate 6** *'The fighting spirit metaphor.'* Drawn by Mr David C. Chin and reproduced with permission.

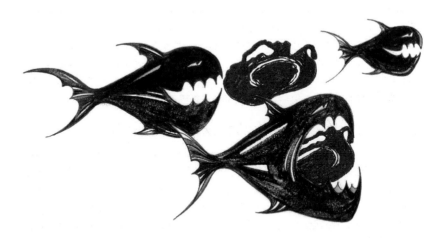

**Colour Plate 7** *'A phagocytic metaphor.'* Drawn by Mr David C. Chin and reproduced with permission.

Exercise may also help to manage symptoms and optimize quality of life for patients with advanced disease. An exercise regimen to help maintain physical functioning and/or attenuate its decline can be developed within the context of the patient's health status, level of function, and personal goals. Functional activities, graduated mobilization, and range of motion exercises may, however, be more appropriate components of the exercise regimen. Determining the optimal regimen in this situation may be best accomplished by an interdisciplinary team that includes a physician, nurse, physical and occupational therapist, dietician, respiratory therapist, and the exercise specialist.

## Alternative forms of exercise

The chosen activity, or type of exercise, should consider the lifestyle needs and preferences of the individual to increase the likelihood of enjoyment and adherence (Courneya *et al.* 2004). Alternative forms of exercise such as dance, Tai Chi Chuan, and Yoga, though less studied, may be preferred over traditional modes. Dance, Tai Chi Chuan, and Yoga may serve to improve flexibility as well as balance and agility (ACSM 2006). A recent study examining dance as an intervention for breast cancer survivors showed substantial improvements in quality of life following the dance movement program (Sandel *et al.* 2005). Tai Chi Chuan is a low-to-moderate intensity form of exercise that has been shown to improve quality of life and self-esteem in breast cancer survivors (Mustian *et al.* 2006). A recent review of the benefits of Yoga for patients with cancer and cancer survivors suggests that it may improve sleep quality, mood, stress, cancer-related symptoms, and overall quality of life (Bower *et al.* 2005). Although exercise intensity is more difficult to control in the class setting, the social interaction may provide motivation and support and improve exercise adherence.

## Precautions and contraindications to exercise

In the design and implementation of exercise programs for cancer survivors, safety must be a priority. Clinical evaluation of the cancer survivor prior to each training session is necessary to rule out underlying instability and/or to identify any deterioration in clinical status. Cancer survivors suffering from ongoing side effects may require closer supervision and monitoring. At minimum, monitoring of blood pressure, heart rate, and vital signs should be performed prior to, several times during, and following the sessions to ensure normal response to, and adequate recovery from, the exercise. Overall, individual medical considerations must be taken into account to ensure that safe and enjoyable exercise training is established. Table 13.3 outlines some of the important cancer-related contraindications that must be taken into account when planning an exercise program for cancer survivors (Courneya *et al.* 2004).

**Table 13.3** Contraindications to exercise in patients with cancer

♦ Abnormal blood count (e.g., low haemoglobin, neutrophils, and platelets)

♦ Fever

♦ Ataxia/dizziness

♦ Severe dyspnoea

♦ Recent onset of bone pain of unknown origin

♦ Severe nausea/vomiting

♦ Severe weight loss/cachexia

♦ Surgical wounds in early stages of healing

♦ Poor functional status: Karnofsky score ≤ 60

## Maintenance of exercise behaviour

For cancer survivors to maintain the beneficial effects from a supervised exercise program, they should be educated on the benefits of exercise and the risks associated with inactivity. The exercise consultation should include counselling on appropriate goal setting and strategies to overcome barriers to physical activity. Cancer survivors should also be instructed in, and practise, the skills of self-monitoring of exercise intensity. This may include instruction in the use of a heart rate monitor and/or pulse rate measurement and of the Borg scale for rating of perceived exertion (ACSM 2006). Successful transition to self-directed and community-based programs can be facilitated by the support of, and regular follow-up from, cancer exercise professionals.

## Conclusion

Increasing attention has been directed towards survivorship issues for individuals diagnosed with cancer. Preliminary research has shown that appropriately prescribed exercise training programs are associated with low complication rates and numerous beneficial effects.

## References

ACSM (ed) 2006, *ACSM's Guidelines for Exercise Testing and Prescription*. Lippincott Williams & Wilkins, Baltimore.

Ardies, C. 2002, Exercise, cachexia, and cancer therapy: a molecular rationale. *Nutrition & Cancer*, vol. **42**, pp. 143–57.

Armstrong, T. L., Almadrones, M. R. & Gilbert, T. 2005, Chemotherapy-induced peripheral neuropathy, *Oncology Nursing Forum Online*, vol. **32**, pp. 305–11.

Batchelor, T. T., Taylor, L. P., Thaler, H. T., Posner, J. B. & DeAngelis, L. M. 1997, Steroid myopathy in cancer patients, *Neurology*, vol. **48**, pp. 1234–38.

Bouchard, C. & Shepard, R. J. 1994, Physical activity, fitness, and health: the model and key concepts. In *Physical Activity, Fitness, and Health: International Proceedings and Consensus Statement*, (eds) C. Bouchard, R. J. Shepard, & T. Stephens, Human Kinetics, Champaign, IL. pp. 77–88.

Bower, J. E., Woolery, A., Sternlieb, B. & Garet, D. 2005, Yoga for cancer patients and survivors, *Cancer Control*, vol. 12, pp. 165–71.

Brown, J. K., Byers, T., Doyle, C. *et al.* 2003, Nutrition and physical activity during and after cancer treatment: an American Cancer Society guide for informed choices, *CA: A Cancer Journal for Clinicians*, vol. 53, pp. 268–91.

Courneya, K. S., Mackey, J. R. & Rhodes, R. E. 2004, Cancer. In *Clinical Exercise Physiology*, (eds) L. M. Lemura, & S. P. von Duvillard, Lippincott Williams & Wilkins, Philadelphia. pp. 387–404.

Floyd, J. D., Nguyen, D. T., Lobins, R. L. *et al.* 2005, Cardiotoxicity of cancer therapy. *Journal of Clinical Oncology*, vol. 23, pp. 7685–96.

Goodwin, P. J., Ennis, M. & Pritchard, K. I. 1999, Adjuvant treatment and onset of menopause preduct weight gain after breast cancer dianosis. *Journal of Clinical Oncology*, vol. 17, pp. 120–9.

Hall, C. M. & Brody, L. T. 1999, *Therapeutic Exercise: Moving Toward Function*, Lippincott Williams & Wilkins, Philadelphia. p. 707.

Holmes. M. D., Chen, W. Y., Feskanich, D., Kroenke, C. H. & Colditz, G. A. 2005, Physical activity and survival after breast cancer diagnosis, *Journal of the American Medical Association*, vol. 293, pp. 2479–86.

Jones, L. W. & Courneya, K. S. 2002, Exercise counseling and programming preferences of cancer survivors, *Cancer Practice*, vol. 10, pp. 208–15.

Jones, L. W., Courneya, K. S., Vallance, J. K. *et al.* 2004, Association between exercise and quality of life in multiple myeloma cancer survivors, *Supportive Care in Cancer*, vol. 12, pp. 780–8.

McArdle, W. D., Katch, F. I. & Katch, V. L. 2001, *Exercise Physiology*, Lippincott Williams & Wilkins, Baltimore. p. 1158.

McNeely, M. L., Campbell, K. L., Rowe, B. H. *et al.* 2006, Effects of exercise on breast cancer patients and survivors: a systematic review and meta-analysis, *Canadian Medical Association Journal*, vol. 175, pp. 34–41.

Meyerhardt, J. A., Giovannucci, E. L., Holmes, M. D. *et al.* 2006a, Physical activity and survival after colorectal cancer diagnosis, *Journal of Clinical Oncology*, vol. 24, pp. 3527–34.

Meyerhardt, J. A., Heseltine, D., Niedzwiecki, D. *et al.* 2006b, Impact of physical activity on cancer recurrence and survival in patients with stage III colon cancer: findings from CALGB 89803, *Journal of Clinical Oncology*, vol. 24, pp. 3535–41.

Moore, I. M. & Hobbie, W. 2000, Late effects of cancer treatment. In *Cancer Nursing: Principles and Practice* (5th ed), (eds) C. H. Yarbo, M. H. Frogge, M. Goodman and S. L. Groenwald. pp. 597–615. Jones and Bartlett, Boston MA.

Mustian, K. M., Katula, J. A. & Zhao, H. 2006, A pilot study to assess the influence of Tai Chi Chuan on functional capacity among breast cancer survivors, *The Journal of Supportive Oncology*, vol. 4, pp. 139–45.

Portenoy, R. K. & Itri, L. M. 1999, Cancer-related fatigue: guidelines for evaluation and management, *The Oncologist*, vol. 4, pp. 1–10.

Sandel, S. L., Judge, J. O., Landry, N., Faria, L., Ouellette, R. & Majczak, M. 2005, Dance and movement program improves quality-of-life measures in breast cancer survivors, *Cancer Nursing*, vol. **28**, no. 4, pp. 301–9.

Schmitz, K. H., Holtzman, J., Courneya, K. S. *et al.* 2005, Controlled physical activity trials in cancer survivors: a systematic review and meta-analysis *Cancer Epidemiology, Biomarkers & Prevention*, vol. **14**, pp. 1588–95.

Stevinson, C., Lawlor, D. A. & Fox, K. A. 2004, Exercise interventions for cancer patients: systematic review of controlled trials, *Cancer Causes and Control*, vol. **15**, pp. 1035–56.

Yeager, K. A., McGuire, D. B. & Sheidler, V. R. 2000, Assessment of cancer pain. In *Cancer Nursing: Principles and Practice*, (eds) C. H. Yarbo, M. H. Frogge, M. Goodman & S. L. Groenwald. Jones and Bartlett, Sudbury, MA.

Chapter 14

# Group support

Barbara Lubrano di Ciccone, Tiffany D Floyd, and David W Kissane

## Summary

Group support allows patients to address cancer-related concerns while also receiving emotional support from others with similar experiences. Such social support is known to act as a buffer against the negative effects of stress. Many types of psychosocial group interventions are available to patients and their families, so it is important to first draw distinctions between them and what they aim to offer. Although groups vary in terms of the specific objectives that are emphasized, in this context they all share the overall goal of helping patients to cope more effectively with the physical, emotional, social, and spiritual sequelae of cancer and its treatment.

## Types of psychosocial group intervention (Table 14.1)

### Psychoeducational groups

The primary goals of psychoeducational groups are to educate patients and improve their abilities to cope with the disease. These groups are usually short term and follow a pre-determined agenda. The role of the group leader is much like that of an instructor in a classroom, providing educational information and assigning exercises for participants to complete as 'homework'. Psychoeducational groups for cancer provide education about cancer and its treatment and training in a variety of stress management and relaxation techniques, such as guided imagery and progressive muscle relaxation. Other useful skills such as problem solving, assertive communication, and constructive thinking may also be taught (Fobair 1997). Learning more about cancer is an important means of increasing self-efficacy for both coping with cancer-related distress (Weis 2003) and participating in the medical environment (Cella and Yellen 1993).

**Table 14.1** Comparison of different types of group interventions for patients with cancer

| | Psychoeducational groups | Psychotherapy groups | Community support groups |
|---|---|---|---|
| **Aim of the intervention** | Improved ability to cope with symptoms of cancer-related distress | Improved psychological well-being and interpersonal relationships | Social support |
| **Mechanism(s) of change** | Increased knowledge | Increased insight and intrapersonal coping resources | Social support |
| **Content of sessions** | Determined by group leader | Determined by group members | Determined by group members |
| **Role of group leader** | Tutorial; very active and directive | Active, gently directive or strategic | Minimally active; non-authoritative |
| **Requisite training of group leader** | Some education and training required about cancer; can be professional or semi-professional | Typically a trained professional (e.g., psychiatrist, psychologist, social worker) | Other support groups: some knowledge of cancer and group processes |
| **Length of group** | Typically short-term | Either short- or long-term | Either short- or long-term |
| **Size of group** | Relatively large, as in a class or seminar: 20–100 | Minimum of 5, maximum of 12 | Minimum of 5, maximum of 12 |
| **Open or closed to new members** | Often closed, due to time-limited nature | Open or closed | Open or closed |

## Psychotherapy groups

The goal of group psychotherapy is to help individuals change something about themselves in order to improve their psychological well-being and relationships with others (Weis 2003). In contrast to psychoeducational groups, psychotherapy groups typically work with patients for a longer term, with their content determined by the group members. The role of the leader is to ensure that patients explore maladaptive thoughts, feelings, and behaviour patterns. They are generally divided into groups for patients with either early stage or advanced cancer, which allows patients to discuss their particular fears and concerns, as well as relationships with healthcare providers (Weis 2003). Common theoretical frameworks used in group psychotherapy include cognitive, existential, and supportive-expressive.

The aim of cognitive therapies is to help people identify their automatic negative thoughts and assist in modifying unhelpful beliefs and accompanying maladaptive behaviour patterns. The interventionist helps develop specific skills for each problem, such as managing and reducing stress, altering thoughts that increase depression, and promoting adaptive strategies that optimize coping (Fobair 1997).

Existential and supportive-expressive groups allow individuals to openly express fears and concerns in a supportive atmosphere. Some degree of cognitive shift invariably follows as people discover new meaning in their circumstances and talk about emotions that are directly linked to common existential challenges. Such therapies stress the idea of taking responsibility for personal choices, actualizing one's unique potential, acknowledging one's ultimate aloneness and mortality, and searching for a sense of personal meaning. Most patients, at one or more points during the course of their illness, will arrive at the question 'Why me?'. The lack of a definitive answer can lead to profound discomfort and individuals are often forced to re-evaluate their previously held beliefs and values (Spiegel and Classen 2000). Confronting issues of mortality is viewed as an important means of alleviating patients' fears about death and dying.

## Community support groups

The primary aim of support groups is to help individuals develop a sense of belonging through participation in the process of mutual support and sharing common experiences, difficulties, and resources with one another. They do not aim to change people, whether through knowledge, skills, or insight. The leader is typically less active or directive than with other types of groups and may, in fact, only intervene in the service of promoting cohesion and/or to provide structure (Cella and Yellen 1993). Support groups diminish stigma and social isolation, build self-esteem, reduce anxiety, and increase patients' confidence in participating in the medical decision-making process.

# Creation of the group

## Selection of the group leader

### Skills and training

Selection of an appropriate group leader is determined by the type of group being created. Professionally trained leaders are prepared to handle the range of content and emotions likely to arise during the course of sessions and to provide appropriate referrals when necessary. Psychotherapy groups are almost invariably led by a mental health professional (e.g. psychiatrist, psychologist, or social worker) who has received extensive training and supervision in the conduct of group psychotherapy and works within specific theoretical orientations.

The most important characteristics of group leaders are empathy, attentiveness, warmth, genuineness, and respectfulness (Fobair 1997). They must avoid personal bias in group facilitation and understand group dynamics (Hermann *et al.* 1995). Knowledge about cancer and the psychosocial issues commonly faced by patients and their families is vital (Fobair 1997).

### Single versus co-leaders

Vugia (1991) and Spiegel and Classen (2000) agree that cancer groups should have two facilitators, with the most effective team represented by someone with medical training (e.g. physician or nurse) and someone skilled in group processes (e.g. psychologist or social worker). Benefits of co-leaders include the ability to: (1) have a broader range of knowledge and experience; (2) have one person lead while the other observes reactions of members; and (3) continue with meetings when one leader is away. Having a single leader may be necessary financially and is preferable to having no leader or no group at all (Spiegel and Classen 2000).

## Selection of group members

Key factors to consider in establishing group cohesion include whether patients share the same type of cancer or stage of disease, and socio-demographic characteristics such as gender and race/ethnicity.

### Same or mixed cancer diagnoses

The most common reason for building a group around a single diagnosis is that it will promote group cohesion among members. More detailed information can be provided about the specific cancer and its treatment and patients may feel more comfortable discussing comparable issues. Breast or prostate cancer groups are commonly homogeneous, whereas bone marrow transplant or adolescent groups may need to be heterogeneous for tumour types.

### Early versus late-stage disease

Homogeneity for stage of disease is important lest advanced-stage patients frighten early-stage patients, who may view it as a negative glimpse of what is to come. Other risks include leading early-stage patients to feel that their problems are trivial by comparison, rejecting outliers as different, fearing getting close to someone who might die, and struggling to preserve optimism about the outcome.

When disease progression occurs in an early-stage group, the question of continued membership arises. Removal of the sicker member is cruel when their need for support is heightened and it sends a negative message of conditional support to the other group members (Spiegel and Classen 2000). Although disease progression may induce anxiety in other members, the affected patient can serve as a role model and source of inspiration (Kissane *et al.* 2004).

Moreover, fears of death and dying and how others will cope with their death may be diminished by viewing others going through the process.

### Gender and race/ethnicity

Both males and racial/ethnic minorities tend to be under-represented in cancer groups. For men, reluctance to join may stem from general discomfort in asking for and receiving emotional support. Cellen and Yellen (1993) recommend incorporating more education and specific skill training in order to attract men, while including topics with greater cultural sensitivity might attract more racial and ethnic minorities.

## Group structure and format

### Group size

Groups should generally range from 5 to 12 members, with the optimal suggested size being 8 (Weis 2003). A larger group of 10–12 accommodates absence due to illness and dropouts (Spiegel and Classen 2000).

### Duration and frequency

Groups typically meet once a week and last for 90 minutes (e.g. Vugia 1991). Meeting less than once a week is not advised as it disrupts the flow of the group and reduces cohesion.

### Setting

The venue needs to be accessible, able to accommodate the group, and typically includes hospitals, neighbourhood clinics, community centres, or college campuses. Access to childcare facilities is a worthwhile consideration.

### Contact outside of the group

Whereas contact outside of the group is generally not allowed in non-cancer psychotherapy groups, it is desirable and encouraged within oncology to promote mutual support. Telephone numbers and email addresses are exchanged. Therapists are wise to ask about out-of-group contact to ensure that no individuals are left out of any gatherings arranged.

## Tasks of the group leader

### Preparing patients for group membership

Leaders should meet with each prospective member individually to ensure that they are aware of the goals and purpose of the group, its basic structure, and meeting arrangements. Exploration of patients' expectations, ambivalences, and hopes enables reality testing and clarification of misconceptions.

This allows group leaders to determine if the patients' goals are compatible with those of the group. Reassurance about benefits over potential harms avoids early dropouts. Avoid bringing together patients with disparate goals, age, and social differences (e.g. a single homosexual member in a heterosexual group) that can disrupt group cohesion. Priority should be given to minimizing potential harm to group members and retaining cohesion, rather than meeting size requirements by allowing incompatible members to join. Patients with active psychiatric problems such as psychosis or severe personality disorder may do better in individual therapy.

General maintenance issues and group norms, such as expectations for attendance, arriving on time, communicating an apology if unavailable, and respecting the confidentiality of the group, should be highlighted (Spiegel and Classen 2000). This promotes safety, alleviates initial apprehension, offers reassurance about the professionalism of the process, and lays the foundation for finding commonality with the other group members.

## Culture building

Perhaps the most important task of group leaders is to establish operational norms, also known as 'culture building' (Yalom and Leszcz 1995). Group norms are the implicit and explicit behavioural rules by which the group conducts itself. Close attention must be paid to this issue because group norms will develop from the beginning. Leaders ensure the ethos created is consistent with the goal of providing a supportive, secure environment in which patients feel free to express themselves openly. Some norms are discussed during the initial screening but most develop during the meetings. Examples of norms would be respecting the contribution of others and taking advantage of opportunities to provide support. The group leaders must be aware of any overt or covert counterproductive attitudes and act to reframe these in a more constructive direction. For example, a patient may feel rejection for sharing fears regarding death and dying, particularly if these fears are shared early on in the group, before members have developed a sense of trust and comfort. The group's initial reaction, left unchecked, could create the implicit norm that it is not okay to openly discuss and explore one's deepest fears when this is precisely what the group is for.

Once established, the culture is difficult to change and so therapists need to work actively from the beginning to establish an enabling rather than a restrictive environment.

## Maintaining focus on the cancer

Some social chitchat promotes warmth and connection, but the primary work of the group should focus on cancer. Some level of social sharing can occur outside the group room. While the aim of the group is to provide support to its members, concentrating on coping with cancer is crucial. Individuals dealing with other significant stressors may benefit from supplemental support.

## Common themes

A number of themes will emerge during the sessions—some will be introduced by the group members, whereas others will need to be suggested by the therapists as appropriate (Classen *et al.* 1993). In general, topics introduced by group members (patient-driven topics) will derive directly from physical concerns resulting from cancer or its treatment, like nausea, pain, fatigue, insomnia, or communication with doctors and family. Topics promoted by the therapists (therapist-driven topics), like sexuality, body image, or existential themes, are often more difficult for patients to bring up themselves, and are usually emotionally charged (Holland *et al.* 1998).

Concerns remote from cancer should never be dismissed absolutely, but explored. It is respectful to validate their individual significance as long as the focus is returned to the cancer experience (Spiegel and Classen 2000).

### Lack of control/helplessness

Many patients enter therapy feeling that their situation is unique and this creates in them a sense of isolation, which in turn can foster a sense of helplessness and lack of control. Although the patient may not have control over the reality of cancer, its course, or troublesome side effects from treatment, group therapy will help them process these issues and facilitate expression of emotions, while providing them with a sense of universality (Yalom and Leszcz 1995). Through sharing their concerns and feelings, patients begin to explore how to react to somatic symptoms, face uncertainty about their future, and take control over their lives again (Kissane *et al.* 1997). The role of the therapist is complex and involves empathic listening and reflection about the feelings patients are experiencing, while helping them recall previous coping and adaptation during adversity (Classen *et al.* 1993; Kissane *et al.* 2004).

### Treatment-related concerns

Discussion of treatment, whether chemotherapy, radiotherapy, or surgery, encompasses concerns and fears related to its potential failure, risks, or side effects (Kissane *et al.* 1997; Kissane *et al.* 2004). When the subject of a patient's discussion becomes externally focused on others, the therapist should redirect the concerns to more personal terms (Holland *et al.* 1998). It is beneficial to the group to discuss how to develop strategies to deal with specific side effects such as fatigue or pain, or how other treatment-related problems affect their quality of life and their relationship with family or doctors. This approach will provide patients with a sense of mastery and enhances mature coping with the unpredictable (Kissane *et al.* 1997).

## Self and body image

With improvement in cancer treatment, self and body image change can be the key to address the psychological impact of these bodily 'injuries' (Holland *et al.* 1998). Depending on the type of cancer, patients will confront issues related to physical disfigurement, feeding, voiding, weight change, or sexuality. Body image reintegration is critical to counter embarrassment and shame after head and neck cancer surgery (Dropkin 1999). Many breast cancer survivors describe negative feelings about their bodies, including decreased self-worth and attractiveness, feeling deformed, inadequate, sad, embarrassed, frustrated, and a sense of loss (Ashing-Giwa *et al.* 2004). As group cohesiveness develops, members will be more open to discuss these concerns. Therapists should explore ways in which patients perceived themselves before and after the cancer or its treatment, helping the group understand the magnitude of the impact, identify any negative self-appraisal, challenge it, and thus improve self-confidence (Kissane *et al.* 1997).

## Health beliefs within the group culture

Cultural health beliefs within the group should be addressed in a sensitive manner. Failure to do this will create a sense of exclusion for members whose beliefs differ from those of the group as a whole. Common cultural issues include those related to traditional healing practices and the use of complementary and alternative medicines, communication styles, language barriers, seeking second opinions, and actual or anticipated discrimination (Glanz *et al.* 2003; Ashing-Giwa *et al.* 2004). Some helpful questions to ask the group are 'What things have helped you recover or cope the most?' and 'What is the best way to handle your illness?' (Ashing-Giwa *et al.* 2004). Members bring diverse coping styles, prior experiences, and varied beliefs, thus creating opportunities to learn from each other and discover alternative approaches that could potentially enhance adaptation (Kissane *et al.* 2004).

## Relationships

Cancer and its treatment affect not only the patients but also the social support systems they have established. Fostering healthy relationships enriches life.

### Doctors and other health care professionals

Trust in the patient–doctor relationship becomes vitally important when confronted with a life-threatening disease. In an ideal world, both patients and doctors communicate efficiently and clearly; patients feel free to ask all the necessary questions and the treatment decision making process is shared without conflict. In reality, oftentimes patients feel intimidated, dependent, and powerless in relation to their doctors. Fear about the disease can interfere with hearing the information correctly or fear of the doctor can prevent them from speaking openly (Classen *et al.* 1993). Through the group exploring ways of building collaborative relationships with doctors and other professional staff, members participate more actively in planning their treatment (Kissane *et al.* 1997).

### Effect of illness on family relationships: partners, children

Stress created by the cancer can have negative effects on the stability of patients' relationships, although separation or divorce due to cancer are infrequent (Holland *et al.* 1998). Issues related to perceived wrongs in the past, marital breakdown, concern over money, substance abuse, rivalries between children, and losses due to incidental life events appear in the long-term life of every group (Kissane *et al.* 2004). Family can also be perceived as a source of strain instead of support for women from different cultural backgrounds, particularly when the family members' own coping difficulties impair the provision of needed support (Ashing-Giwa *et al.* 2004). Group therapy allows members to express relationship concerns and helps them improve communication with their families. Children should also be part of family discussions. This will decrease their feelings of confusion and anxiety (Classen *et al.* 1993).

## Existential issues

Few cancer group intervention trials have specifically addressed existential or spiritual themes and outcomes as the main focus (Breitbart 2002). However, 'Why me?' is frequently asked as patients face life-threatening illness, and this question can be a valuable introduction to existential discussion.

Important issues expressed by patients have been represented in the following five items: recognizing that life is at times unfair; recognizing that ultimately there is no escape from some of life's pain and from death; recognizing that no matter how close we get to others, we must still face life alone; facing the basic issues of life and death, living more honestly, and being less caught up in trivialities; and learning to take ultimate responsibility for the way we live, no matter how much guidance and support we get (Yalom and Leszcz 1995).

Religion also comes up as the group discusses existential concerns. In this instance, the role of the group is not to challenge or replace any religious beliefs but to help members better manage the process of living and dying (Spiegel and Classen 2000). The role of therapists is to help members find their own sense of spirituality while assessing its impact on quality of life and health (Cunningham 2005).

## Disruptions to the group

### Difficult members (e.g. monopolizers, silent members, help-rejecters)

The monopolizer is someone who will continuously talk at the expense of other group members. Silences make them anxious and they jump in to speak at every opportunity. If not addressed in a timely and sensitive manner, the fate of the group may be doomed. Therapists may ask the group why they allow and encourage one member to 'carry the burden of the entire meeting?' Fostering a discussion among other members about reasons for their inactivity or passivity will enhance the therapeutic process (Yalom and Leszcz 1995). Another approach looks directly at the monopolizer. Here, therapists keep a close track of the timing and content of the monopolizer's comments, noticing when he or she takes the floor, or changes the topic soon after someone has said something distressing. In this case, a therapist could reflect, 'I am wondering if you felt a need to change the topic to something not so upsetting?' (Classen *et al.* 1993). The goal is not to silence the person but to enable them to talk more about deeply felt personal conflicts. If the therapist attempts to silence the monopolizer, the therapeutic purpose of the group will be lost; the monopolizer will eventually drop out, while the rest of the group might become uncomfortable with the therapists.

The silent member poses the opposite problem. Silence can be a signal of anxiety, fear, and dread of self-disclosure, or varied cultural beliefs. The therapist can comment on the member's silence, express concern, and inquire if it is possible to discuss with the group what makes participation difficult. The therapist's task is not only to change behaviour but to help the patient gain self-knowledge (Yalom and Leszcz 1995).

The help-rejecter, first recognized by Jerome Frank in 1952, is the 'yes, but' patient, who insists on looking for help but is then unable to find someone competent enough to help or understand. In general, the help-rejecter takes pride in the insolubility of his or her problem or receives gratification from being in constant need of help. The group will soon become bored and frustrated by this attitude and the therapist must remain vigilant that this patient does not become estranged from the others.

### Disease progression

Cancer type, stage, and treatment options can influence progression of the disease, which represents a challenge not only for the patient but for the group as a whole. Patients facing disease progression encounter significant emotional distress and have feelings of guilt or failure, with the group being the only safe place to discuss their circumstances openly. They should be discouraged from abandoning the group, whose members might otherwise become demoralized and fearful of eventually facing the same fate (Classen *et al.* 1993). Nevertheless, it can be so frightening for some patients that it may result in their leaving the group (Spiegel and Classen 2000). This is an opportunity to discuss what is most feared and to learn how to cope more actively, managing pain and stress, and receiving emotional support (Holland *et al.* 1998).

## Loss of a group member

The two most common ways that a cancer group loses members is by voluntary dropout or death. Both cause distress to the remaining group and members' concerns should be addressed promptly. If someone leaves because they are frightened of talking about cancer, it is important to address and validate these fears. Group leaders can reiterate that an excellent way of coping is to talk about various ways in which people are affected (Classen *et al.* 1993).

Death of a group member is naturally stressful, causing concern and fear. Group leaders must remain cognizant of this and help patients tolerate their thoughts of death and dying. Paradoxically, openly talking about issues of death and dying will help the group to 'detoxify' these thoughts (Spiegel and Classen 2000).

# Challenges to the group process

This section focuses on issues relevant to the therapist–patient relationship, the termination of care, and barriers to care.

## Transference/countertransference

Transference refers to the perceptions or feelings that the patient develops towards the therapist. Countertransference refers to those that the therapist develops towards the group. Both phenomena can have either positive or negative impact on the group; we focus here on the negative. Transference issues usually present subtly; they can be observed when therapists enter the room. Yalom (1995) notes that: 'the therapist's arrival not only reminds the group of its task but also evokes early constellations of feelings in each member about the adult, the teacher, the evaluator' (p. 193).

When not properly addressed, these phenomena can potentially split the group and transform it into a non-nurturing environment. Transference can also split the therapist into a kind and generous person or a cold and absent one. Several issues intrinsic to the process of cancer groups can be challenging for therapists. For instance, what will the group's reaction be if the therapist does not attend the funeral of a member, is absent at a time perceived as particularly difficult, or is perceived as 'whole' in terms of health and not missing any body parts? Key strategies include identifying differences of opinion within the group, drawing out expressions of ambivalence, nurturing inclusiveness and cohesiveness, and facing existential concerns (Kissane *et al.* 2004). Countertransference also presents a challenge for therapists, especially when two therapists feel differently about the group. Open discussion between co-therapists is worthwhile to nurture a genuine, creative, and conducive environment.

## When the group has to end

Termination can be a challenging time for the group and members should periodically be reminded of the number of sessions remaining. The leaders can help the group identify 'unfinished business', disclose feelings about the loss of the group, and focus on 'future-oriented' reflections, like how their lives have changed and what have they learned about self and others (Kissane *et al.* 1997). Termination can involve a mourning process. There will be some resistance to accepting its end, including anger, and members may bargain with the therapists to continue longer.

These attempts are powerful statements about the importance of the group and therapists should acknowledge this openly, while helping members confront their own feelings about saying good-bye (Classen *et al.* 1993).

## Barriers to care

Patients may encounter barriers to access to care. Although some of these involve practical issues like financial status, insurance coverage, employment, or education, members should be encouraged to voice any concerns and not permit them to become justified reasons for missing sessions. Allowing the group to participate in the solution will create a sense of increased control and cohesiveness.

## Benefits of being in a group

A growing body of evidence suggests that patients who participate in group therapy achieve better coping skills and adaptation (Spiegel and Classen 2000), including improved psychological outcomes in metastatic breast cancer (Goodwin 2005). One early study by Spiegel *et al.* reported extended survival from group therapy but other research has failed to replicate this finding

(Goodwin *et al.* 2001; Kissane *et al.* 2004). Nonetheless, improvement in quality of life has been repeatedly demonstrated and the psychological support received through supportive-expressive group therapy creates an environment in which greater compliance with anti-cancer therapy occurs (Kissane *et al.* 2004).

# References

Ashing-Giwa, K. T., Padilla, G., Tejero, J. *et al.* 2004, Understanding the breast cancer experience of women: a qualitative study of African American, Asian American, Latina and Caucasian cancer survivors, *Psycho-oncology,* vol. **13**, no. 6, pp. 408–28.

Breitbart, W. 2002, Spirituality and meaning in supportive care: spirituality- and meaning-centered group psychotherapy interventions in advanced cancer, *Supportive Care in Cancer,* vol. **10**, no. 4, pp. 272–80.

Cella, D. F. & Yellen, S. B. 1993, Cancer support groups: the state of the art, *Cancer Practice,* vol. **1**, no. 1, pp. 56–61.

Classen, C., Diamond, S., Soleman, A., Fobair, P., Spira, J. & Spiegel, D. 1993, Brief supportive-expressive therapy for women with primary breast cancer: a treatment manual. Psychosocial Treatment Laboratory, Breast Cancer Intervention Project, Stanford School of Medicine - Department of Psychiatry and Behavioral Sciences.

Cunningham, A. J. 2005, Integrating spirituality into a group psychological therapy program for cancer patients, *Integrative Cancer Therapies,* vol. **4**, no. 2, pp. 178–86.

Dropkin, M. J. 1999, Body image and quality of life after head and neck cancer surgery, *Cancer Practice,* vol. **7**, no. 6, pp. 309–13.

Fobair, P. 1997, Cancer support groups and group therapies: Part II, process organizational, leadership, and patient issues, *Journal of Psychosocial Oncology,* vol. **15**, pp. 123–47.

Glanz, K., Croyle, R. T., Chollette, V. Y. & Pinn, V. W. 2003, Cancer-related health disparities in women, *American Journal of Public Health,* vol. **93**, no. 2, pp. 292–8.

Goodwin, P. J. 2005, Support groups in advanced breast cancer, *Cancer,* vol. **104**, pp. 2596–601.

Goodwin, P. J., Leszcz, M., Ennis, M. *et al.* 2001, The effect of group psychosocial support on survival in metastatic breast cancer *New England Journal of Medicine,* vol. **345**, no. 24, pp. 1719–26.

Hermann, J. F., Cella, D. F. & Robinovitch, A. 1995, Guidelines for support group programs, *Cancer Practice,* vol. **3**, no. 2, pp. 111–3.

Holland, J. C., Breitbart, W., Jacobsen, P. B. *et al.,* (eds) 1998, *Psycho-Oncology.* Oxford University Press, New York.

Kissane, D. W., Bloch, S., Miach, P., Smith, G. C., Seddon, A. & Keks, N. 1997, Cognitive-existential group therapy for patients with primary breast cancer - techniques and themes, *Psycho-oncology,* vol. **6**, no. 1, pp. 25–33.

Kissane, D. W., Grabsch, B., Clarke, D. M. *et al.* 2004, Supportive-expressive group therapy: the transformation of existential ambivalence into creative living while enhancing adherence to anti-cancer therapies, *Psycho-oncology,* vol. **13**, no. 11, pp. 755–68.

Kissane, D. W., Love, A., Hatton, A. *et al.* 2004, Effect of cognitive-existential group therapy on survival in early-stage breast cancer, *Journal of Clinical Oncology,* vol. **22**, no. 21, pp. 4255–60.

Spiegel, D. & Classen, C. 2000, *Group therapy for cancer patients: a research-based handbook of psychosocial care*. Basic Books, New York.

Vugia, H. D. 1991, Support groups in oncology: building hope through the human bond, *Journal of Psychosocial Oncology*, vol. **9**, pp. 89–107.

Weis, J. 2003, Support groups for cancer patients, *Supportive Care in Cancer*, vol. **11**, no. 12, pp. 763–8.

Yalom, I. D. & Leszcz, M. 1995, *The Theory and Practice of Group Psychotherapy*. Basic Books, New York.

Chapter 15

# Healing

Diane O'Connell

## Summary

The practice of healing can take many different forms but always involves the focusing of energy with a healing intent. This chapter gives an overview of healing: what it is, who practises it, the benefits it can bring, and the problems occasionally experienced. It includes case studies to illustrate how healing can be used for patients with cancer. Each person takes what he or she needs from the healing—this may mean relaxation, feeling supported, alleviation of symptoms, and/or awareness of a spiritual dimension to life. Sometimes, it is about the quality of the dying process and 'healing into death'.

## Introduction

How does healing differ from the multitude of other natural therapies that abound in the realm of cancer care? Because it appears on the surface so ethereal and other-worldly, it is easy to overlook this ancient art and science. We could say that the 'healing intent' that lies behind both conventional and natural forms of therapy is not something that is easily demonstrable in a concrete way; yet, is widely understood and accepted as valid. We could hypothesize that it derives from non-visible dimensions—the wellspring of the varied forms of healing itself.

Today, healing is practised in every country in the world, especially in England where we have well over 20,000 registered healers, making it one of the largest complementary therapies in the country. Healing has been continually practised down the ages and many traditions speak of the Shaman, or Medicine Man/Woman, who demonstrated from pre-historic times the ability to act as an intermediary and bring healing and harmony. An Egyptian papyrus at least 3500 years old mentions the laying-on-of-hands for pain relief.

## So, what is healing?

One of the most succinct definitions is given by Benor (1992): 'Healing is any systematic, purposeful intervention by a person purporting to help another living thing (person, animal, plant or other living system) or part thereof to change via the sole process of focused intention or via hand contact or passes'. Other defi-nitions may attempt to define the source of the healing energy or intent. The word healing derives from ancient Germanic and English roots and means 'to make whole' (Benor 2004) and this is the intent of the healer. It is often said that healing is a process and not an event and may not produce a 'cure' in the usually accepted sense. A common way that healers explain their work is that they put out their intention, step aside, and allow a flow of healing energy to pass through them to the recipient ('healee'). Healers use their hands to direct this energy either by touching the person (laying on of hands) or working just above the body. The energy or hands take them to the place that needs healing and it is there that they focus their intent. Healers often experience sensations in their hands such as heat, cold, tingling, or heaviness.

There are two main methods of healing:

+ Contact healing where the client is present

+ Distant healing where the client is absent

Healing can incorporate a variety of other techniques such as prayer, invoca-tion, affirmation, visualization, sound, colour, and crystals.

Descriptions of what healers do are likely to challenge the belief systems of a rational or scientific mind. Therefore, healing is often looked upon with scepti-cism and any benefit is explained by the 'placebo effect'. In some instances, this could well be the case—subjective matters are very hard to prove, given the limited knowledge we have regarding the power of the mind. However, as Harlow (2003) comments: 'There is a tendency to dismiss the placebo effect as somehow improper, as a form of therapeutic cheating. We should seek rather to explore how the placebo effect actually works and how it differs from the effect of healing'.

There is a large body of anecdotal evidence as well as many scientific studies which suggest that both contact and distant healing do work. Benor (1992) states that there have been more controlled studies on healing than on all the other complementary therapies combined. He also asks the question 'Is there adequate research to confirm the hypothesis that spiritual healing is effective?' and answers with a resounding 'Yes'.

## The journey of the healer

The majority of practitioners in England call themselves Spiritual Healers and work by invoking agents such as God, Christ, or spirit guides to support their healing intent. Others call themselves Energy Workers, Energy Healers, or Reiki Healers because they see life as the interplay of energy and will work to balance the energetic system of the client with healing energy channelled through them and manipulated in different ways. They experience the human body surrounded by an energy system called an aura, sometimes considered to be an electromagnetic field that has qualities of consciousness emanating from the physical, emotional, mental, and spiritual aspects of the client.

Healers who combine their healing with other skills may call themselves, for example, Colour Healers, Sound Healers, or Crystal Healers. In America, the term Therapeutic Touch is widely used instead of healing and has found favour in hospitals and other mainstream environments because it approaches the subject from a less metaphysical point of view. There is also the Healing Ministry, which is carried out within the Christian and Spiritualist Churches as well as other religions. The healing is carried out by the priest and/or lay people and involves prayer and invocation as well as the laying on of hands.

Healers vary considerably in their approach, as Benor (2004) states: 'Healers' beliefs and techniques are as varied as human experience and imagination can make them'. This makes healing a very difficult complementary therapy to explain or understand as it challenges the belief systems of many. There is, however, one factor that all healers have in common and that is their healing intent: '…it didn't seem to matter what method you (the healer) used, as long as you held an intention for a patient to heal' (McTaggert 2001). This is a very powerful statement as it implies that if we hold the intention for healing it has an effect whether we are a healer or not. The intent the healer holds is for the Highest Good of the patient.

Healers could, therefore, be described as individuals who have developed the ability to focus their healing intent. This can express itself in many different ways depending on the belief system, lifestyle, and background culture of the person concerned. Some healers have, over the centuries, demonstrated instantaneous healings that might be called miracles. However, the majority tend to produce more gradual results over a period of time in which they help and support the client through their healing crisis. Because cancer treatment also usually takes place over an extended period, the alliance formed between healer and healee can be very significant in the patient's journey and often helps in the parallel journey being made with conventional approaches.

A healer's development may occur in many different ways:

- Having the natural gift of healing
- Being told they are a healer and developing the skill
- Going through their own healing crises
- Developing healing as part of their spiritual/religious practice
- Seeing healing as a complementary therapy and a vocational pathway

## Benefits of healing for health professionals to consider

- Does not conflict with orthodox treatments
- Patients routinely report a sense of well-being and relaxation, feeling calm, safe, and nurtured
- Patients are not required to give a detailed medical history
- Patients often feel immediate benefit
- Patients have been observed to suffer fewer side-effects from chemotherapy than the norm
- Recovery from surgery is often quicker
- Helps patients to remain balanced emotionally and psychologically and live each day as it comes
- Listening ear of the healer can enhance patients' well-being
- Patients do not necessarily need to expend energy during treatment or undergo uncomfortable or embarrassing techniques/procedures
- Patients do not have to be present
- No serious side-effects have been found
- Low cost
- No purchase of medicines necessary
- Significant number of practitioners (many of whom come from an ethical standpoint and are not reliant on this for their livelihoods) with bench-marked standards in place for training and supervision
- Professional associations with codes of conduct and disciplinary procedures
- Most healers are covered by good-quality professional treatment insurance (very low cost because of claims record practically non-existent)
- There is quite a body of research that has shown definite (but as yet unexplainable) beneficial effect from healing, which cannot be attributable merely to placebo

We have considered the benefits; is there any potential downside?

## Problems occasionally experienced

- Unrealistic expectations of the treatment or therapist
- Although it can work without patients' knowing, there are issues of consent especially with distant healing—although this is normally conducted in a spirit of goodwill

- If patients are very resistant (for religious, cultural, or other reasons), this can limit the effectiveness of the healing
- Some people do not like being touched and although there are many styles that do not touch the body, there are some that do
- It is agreed that most, if not all, therapeutic interventions carry a degree of uncertainty

## Healing for patients with cancer

Patients suffering from any type of cancer may seek healing at any stage of their disease:

- After initial diagnosis
- During conventional treatment
- After the cancer has returned, maybe after months or years
- Having been told they have only a short time to live

Although the healing intent will be the same for all patients, the way the healer works will be unique for each. Healing is a holistic therapy and works on the whole person physically, emotionally, mentally, and spiritually. A cancer diagnosis for most people is a shocking experience and that shock can resonate on all levels. The patient with cancer has to deal with the actual symptoms of disease, the trauma of the diagnosis, and the reaction of family and friends. Healing can help the patient to regain emotional and mental balance and therefore support him/her in coping with their situation.

Krieger (1993) states 'there are several consistent and highly reliable results of Therapeutic Touch':

- Relaxation
- Pain reduction
- Accelerated healing process
- Alleviation of psychosomatic illness

These same responses are commonly experienced in all the different styles of healing and all of them will help the patient with cancer. The Bristol Cancer Help Centre (now Penny Brohn Cancer Care) recommends healing to their patients and Dr Rosy Daniel, their former Medical Director, says in her book on cancer prevention (2001) 'The beauty of healing is that you do not have to think, talk or do any work at all. The only requirement is to be receptive to the healing energy. This is a bit like lying back and enjoying the sun or soaking in a warm bath'. This makes healing a very supportive and beneficial therapy for all patients with cancer, especially those very ill ones who feel they do not have the energy to participate actively. Patients who are unable to go to see a healer can receive distant healing or the healer will visit the patient at home or in hospital.

# Case histories

## Julia

Julia came to see me with a diagnosis of cancer of the colon, which had spread into surrounding organs including the liver. She had been told that she had only 3 months to live. She was shocked by the situation she was in, being only 39 and having three children under 8 years. I went to Julia's home to give her healing weekly. She found the healing helped her to relax, calming her thinking and emotions as well as giving her more physical stamina. After 3 months, the doctors at hospital felt the chemotherapy was working and they decided to continue it for another 3 months. It was during this phase of the treatment that Julia experienced a bright white light fill her body during the healing and as it left she knew it had taken the cancer with it. She did not tell me of this incident until months later. However, she did tell a very close friend because she felt that if things had changed she wanted someone to know of the experience when it had happened.

Six months after her original diagnosis Julia was well and had tolerated two courses of chemotherapy with few side-effects. When the scans came through again the doctors felt that it was possible to operate and to their amazement they found there was no cancer in the colon, only thickening and a grade 1 cancer in one of the ovaries that they removed. There were three small patches of cancer in the liver but other than that she was clear. Julia was delighted. There was no sign of secondaries anywhere else in the body. When Julia was telling me about this, she told me of her experience months before of how she felt that the cancer had left her body during the healing. When she told her friend about the findings, the friend said well we knew it had all gone months ago!

Although we cannot definitely say that this was all due to the healing I think it is true that the healing working alongside conventional treatment made a big difference in Julia's recovery from cancer. She herself feels that it has been a great support and wishes to continue having healing on a regular basis.

## John

Not all clients have such a wonderful remission as Julia. Working with patients who have terminal cancer is very challenging for both healer and healee. The healing is given to support them at all levels so they are able to approach their death as well as possible. One such client was John who, when he heard he had cancer, felt that this was his time to die. He put his affairs in order and died very quickly after the diagnosis, far sooner than expected. He had no sense that he should fight the disease or make changes; he just felt it was his time. The healing was to support him and to allow his death to be as peaceful as possible.

# Paul

Paul is the son of a colleague of mine, who was training to be a healer at the time her son became sick. This is Paul's description:

'My first experience of healing was an incredibly powerful one. I was 18 and in a hospital isolation unit, half way through my first course of chemotherapy treatment for acute leukaemia. I was extremely ill: my immune system had collapsed, my body was not producing red blood cells and I was being kept alive on blood transfusions and prophylactic antibiotics and antifungal medications. I had an infection in the bone of my upper jaw and nasal cavities that made my face swell up causing me immense pain. I was also suffering from the effects of the chemotherapy. As well as the nausea and vomiting, the chemo felt that it was burning me inside—which of course it was. I could not eat or sleep, the whole of my being felt like it was on fire, and I was writhing, desperate to get out of my body and away from the pain, but also aware that I had to stay there and bear it, in order to keep living.

I dimly remember that into this hell came two people, a man and a woman. They brought with them an air of calm and peace. They stood either side of my bed and gave me healing. I remember vague images, thoughts and feelings; the long slow sounds of their deliberate breathing, like waves; the palpable feeling of their attention on me, like hands holding me; the feeling of hands moving over me; the distinct difference in the male and female energy, one on either side of me, dark and like earth and sky, and the balance this gave; a cooling and calming feeling, like waves on a stormy sea settling down in me. Notice how the imagery here turns from fire to water. That is what it felt like. Soothing and settling. I felt as though my bewildered and scattered energies had been helped back into some sort of alignment, like reorganizing the last few survivors of an army back into ranks to face the rest of the battle. I was still in a desperate place, but I felt less teased out, more solid, less scrambled, more real, and more prepared to face what was coming. They left and I slept properly for the first time in several days'.

Paul's mother continued to help him with direct healing throughout his illness and subsequent courses of chemotherapy, radiotherapy, and bone marrow transplant. Paul comments that 'most of the time I was quite spaced out and unable to interact much in the material world. I think the healing reached me in the place I had withdrawn into and provided an extra dimension of care and support that complemented and balanced the physical medical treatment I was having. As my father put it, "witches and garage mechanics". Balance. Holism'.

When Paul's mother told me that he had been diagnosed with leukaemia, he and his family were immediately put on the distant healing list and as he was so ill they received healing daily for many weeks. I asked Paul's mother what her experience of the healing was and she said, 'I guess the healing process is containing and empowering for the carer. It helps affirm what CAN be done, rather than being overwhelmed by fear and despair. I don't believe it sets up false hopes. It does allow a spiritual knowing and being to be present which holds the all too volatile personal in such crises or endurances'.

Both Paul and Julia are alive and well 2 years later.

## Where healers practise

With over 20,000 healers registered with different professional organizations throughout the UK, healing is a well-established complementary therapy. Healers can be accessed as follows:

*Healing centres*: These are often run by healing organizations. Healers meet, usually once a week and new clients are allocated a healer. In some centres, there is a rota of healers, most of whom are volunteers. These centres usually work on a donation basis and sometimes the healing is free.

*Distant healing groups*: Healers meet, usually once a week and have a list of people who want healing. The healing may have been asked for on behalf of the patient by a relative. The patient will be given a time when the healing will be sent and asked to relax and be open to receiving the energy. Feedback to the group is invited. Again, this service can be free or by donation.

*Private practice*: Some healers see the client for half an hour and just give healing and others take an hour in which they spend time talking to the client before and after the healing. Further skills may be involved, such as listening and feedback using counselling skills, or teaching self-healing techniques and visualizations to help empower the client. Healers who work in private practice will often send distant healing to clients between sessions to offer support. Healers working in this way will either charge or work for a donation.

*National Health Service (NHS)*: Healing was the first complementary therapy to be accepted by the NHS, with healers being allowed to visit patients in hospital. Healers now work in some doctors' surgeries as well.

*Spiritualist churches*: The healing takes place within a religious context and often the healing is freely given to all during the service.

*Churches and other faiths*: The healing ministry within the Christian Church and other religions is carried out by the priests, officers, and lay members. The healing is carried out through prayer and/or the laying on of hands.

All these different approaches enable patients with cancer to receive healing in a way that suits their needs and belief systems.

## Standards

People suffering from life-threatening illnesses are very vulnerable and need to know that the healer they are going to see is accredited and of an appropriate standard. In many countries of the world, healers belong to healing organizations, which have their own standards of training, competence, code of practice, and in some cases, insurance. In the UK, for example, there are many healing organizations that accredit their standard of training and through them clients can check whether a healer is registered. The Internet is a valuable resource for finding out more.

## Conclusion

Over more than 30 years of practice, I have worked with patients with cancer at all stages of their journey, using both contact and distant healing, and my experience has shown me that healing does made a difference. Some patients experience help with their symptoms and the unwanted effects of conventional treatment. Others feel supported on an emotional and mental level to come to terms with the situation they find themselves in, and some may become aware of a spiritual dimension in their lives for the first time. In all cases, they have found benefit and support.

The world of healing has much to offer cancer sufferers. Through the millennia, this form of therapy has given benefit to millions of people. Not all patients with cancer survive their illness but their quality of life and sense of well-being can be enhanced by the experience of healing.

## References

Benor, D. J. 1992, *Healing Research Volume One*. Helix Editions Ltd., Deddington, Oxfordshire.

Benor, D. J. 2004, *Consciousness Bioenergy and Healing*. Wholistic Healing Publications, Medford, New Jersey.

Daniel, R. 2001, *The Cancer Prevention Book*. Simon & Shuster UK Ltd., London.

Harlow, T. 2003, In *Healing Intention and Energy Medicine*, (eds) W. B. Jonas, C. C. Crawford, Churchill Livingstone, London.

Krieger, D. 1993, *Accepting your Power to Heal*. Bear and Company, Santa Fe, New Mexico.

McTaggart, L. 2001, *The Field*. Harper Collins, London.

## Useful web sites

www.collegeofhealing.org
www.councilforhealing.org
www.therapeutic-touch.org
www.ukhealers.info
www.wholistichealingresearch.com

Chapter 16

# Herbal medicine

Doreen Oneschuk, Jawaid Younus, and
Heather Boon

## Summary

Many patients with cancer make use of herbal therapies in the hope of an
anti-cancer effect, to decrease cancer-related symptoms, and/or to improve
quality of life. Herbal natural health products are available in several forms
including teas, tinctures, and capsules. Product regulation is country
dependent. In dealing with herbal products, it is important for healthcare
practitioners to be aware of product quality and standardization issues.
In addition, practitioners must be alert to the potential for interactions
with other medications, chemotherapy, and radiation therapy. Practitioners
should acquire knowledge and skills so that they can effectively counsel
patients with cancer who choose to use herbal products. The evidence base
for five common herbs is discussed in this chapter.

## Introduction

The use of herbs for medicinal purposes dates back to the time of unwritten
records. Many herbs can be traced back to the ancient Egyptian and
Mesopotamian civilizations and subsequently to Greco-Roman times. Given
that herbal knowledge has always been part of general culture (Porter 1997),
it is not surprising that herbal therapies even today continue to hold the interest of patients, including those with cancer. There is a widespread assumption
that it must be safe to take something that comes from nature and that herbs
will have gentler effects compared with conventional medicines. Although
many herbs are quite safe and some have demonstrated anti-cancer effects in
cell cultures, further research is necessary to assess their safety and efficacy
when ingested by humans.

Herbal preparations are commonly used by patients with cancer in various
stages of their illness trajectory (Boon et al. 2000). By strict definition, herbs

are 'non-woody, seed-producing plants that die at the end of growing season'. Herbal products can comprise the whole plant as well as leaves, flowers, stems, seeds, roots, fruit, bark, or other parts used for medicinal effects, fragrance, or food flavouring. The three most common forms of medicinal herbs are herbal teas, tinctures, and capsules. Herbal teas are the traditional preparation of Europe and most Asian countries, tinctures are liquid alcoholic extracts taken in the form of drops, and capsules contain dried, powdered, or freeze-dried herb or herb extracts. Herbal products are also available in many other dosage forms such as chewable tablets, lozenges, lollipops, creams, essential oils, and volatile oil preparations, and as complements of vitamin–mineral supplements and food concentrate preparations.

Herbs are an important component of many different traditional systems of medicine such as traditional Chinese medicine (TCM) and Ayurveda. Herbal therapies are frequently used with or after conventional interventions. They may be used as part of a holistic regimen to drain the body of 'toxins', to strengthen the immune system, to improve quality of life, and/or to decrease cancer-related symptoms.

## Herbal quality, contamination, adulteration, potency, strength, and standardization

A critical factor affecting both the safety and efficacy of a herbal remedy is its quality. Quality includes correct identification, prevention of contamination or adulteration, as well as accuracy when describing the potency or strength of the product including standardization to specific 'active' principles where appropriate. Ensuring the correct botanical identity is an essential first step (McCutcheon and Beatty 2000). This includes use of the Latin binomial and authority to rigorously identify a given botanical product as well as the need to independently assess any plant products used in clinical trials. Ideally, consumers should be able to find this information on product labels to allow them to compare product selections with those used in clinical studies.

The unintentional inclusion of material from the wrong plant part, the wrong plant species, or other foreign material is referred to as 'contamination'. Microbial, pesticide and herbicide, heavy metal, and radioactive contamination can occur. The intentional addition of either another herb or foreign substance for reasons such as increasing the weight or potency, or to decrease cost, is referred to as 'adulteration'. The most common forms of product adulteration include the addition of inexpensive materials such as starch, lead, or cheap herbs to increase weight. The form of adulteration that poses the greatest health risks is the addition of undeclared pharmaceuticals to herbal products (McCutcheon and Beatty 2000).

The method of preparation is a critical factor in determining the chemical make-up of strength, stability, and bioavailability of a herbal product (McCutcheon and Beatty 2000). Standardization is an attempt to ensure comparable and replicable doses of compounds (usually, but not always, active compounds) in each dose of a herbal preparation. Representative samples of the same plant species can have varying compositions, including variations in the chemical compounds responsible for target biological activities. The variation in composition may be due to growing the species in different soils; differing climatic conditions from one year to the next; diurnal variations in phytochemical content; genetic variability within a single herb species; age or maturity of the plant; harvesting, drying, and storage conditions; and/or solvent and extraction conditions (McCutcheon and Beatty 2000; Block *et al.* 2004). Standardization of the extracts entails a procedure of extraction and concentration of varying batches of plant material to produce a herbal product with a consistent level of the active compound(s) (Block *et al.* 2004).

## Regulation

Regulation of herbal products varies dramatically around the world, from strict licensing that models conventional drug regulatory processes to virtually no regulation at all. The European Commission, which governs the European Union, has recently promulgated a draft directive on the licensing of traditional herbal preparations. If accepted, this proposal will compel all members of the European Union to introduce a simplified procedure for these preparations so that they can receive a 'traditional use' registration without the need to present data on efficacy from randomized trials. The simplified licensing approach allows a premarketing assessment of the quality and safety of a product and facilitates postmarketing surveillance and product recalls. It does not guarantee efficacy in the same stringent ways that the approval process for conventional medications does (Benzi and Ceci 1997).

Most herbal products in the United States are considered dietary supplements and meet the standards set forth in the 1994 Dietary Supplement and Health Education Act. They are marketed without prior approval of their efficacy and safety by the Food and Drug Administration (De Smet 2002). Herbs that are used in Canada to prevent, diagnose, or treat disease or to maintain/promote health and that are endorsed for self-care purposes are regulated as natural health products (NHPs). A full range of health claims including structure–function, risk-reduction, and therapeutic, or treatment claims are allowed for NHPs, provided that acceptable evidence exists to support the claim. All NHPs require premarket approval by the Natural

Health Products Directorate of Health Canada. In addition, all Canadian manufacturers, packagers, labellers, and importers must have site licenses and meet the good manufacturing standards outlined in the regulations (http://www.hc-sc.gc.ca/dhp-mps/prodnatur/index_e.html).

## Safety issues, drug interactions, and interactions with chemotherapy and radiation

A major cause of concern is the potential for herbs to interact with prescription drugs. The combined use of herbs and anti-cancer drugs may increase or reduce the effects of either component, possibly resulting in clinically important interactions. Synergistic therapeutic effects may complicate the dosing regimen of long-term medications or lead to unfavourable toxicity. Herbal preparations may interact with conventional anti-cancer drugs at various anatomic or physiological sites, changing the rate of elimination or the amount of drug absorbed (De Smet 2002). When a herb is given in combination with anti-cancer drugs, all aspects of pharmacokinetics might be affected, including absorption (resulting in altered absorption rate or oral bioavailability), distribution (mostly cased by protein-binding displacement), metabolism, and excretion. Many known drug interactions are due to changes in metabolic routes related to altered expression or functionality of cytochrome P450 (CYP) enzymes (Kivisto et al. 1995). Extraction of anti-cancer drugs by extensive metabolism in the gut wall and/or liver during first pass is another potential mechanism involved in suspected interactions for various agents (Kruijtzer et al. 2002; Sparreboom et al. 2004).

Free radicals and reactive oxygen species mediate antitumour activity as well as adverse effects of some conventional agents. Antioxidants may limit adverse effects but could also theoretically diminish antitumour efficacy. Because the generation of free radicals is central to the cytotoxic effects of radiation, the theoretical risk that antioxidants might diminish efficacy of radiation therapy (RT) is particularly high. Some chemotherapeutic agents may also rely on free radicals and reactive oxygen species as mediators of cytotoxicity.

Studies that have tested the combination of non-prescription antioxidants with these 'high-risk' conventional therapies have yielded mixed results. Most randomized control trials (RCTs) have not demonstrated significant differences in efficacy with concurrent antioxidant administration. Although no RCTs have yet shown inhibition of radiation efficacy by antioxidants, inhibition has been noted in two animal studies. Other chemotherapeutic agents do not seem to depend on free radicals and reactive oxygen species for their therapeutic efficacy. These agents might be considered theoretically at lower risk for potential inhibition by antioxidants. However, unexpected interactions may result if either potentiation or inhibition of these 'low-risk' agents occurs. Even if a specific agent is known to generate free radicals, it is not always clear that these radicals play an essential role in antitumour activity. In summary, the limited data to date suggest that concurrent administration of antioxidants may result in either potentiation or inhibition of RT and chemotherapy. The outcome of any given pairing of an antioxidant with a conventional regimen is difficult to predict from theoretical models (Weiger *et al.* 2002).

With regard to herb–drug interactions, some herbs possess antiplatelet activity, adversely interact with corticosteroids and central nervous system depressant drugs, have gastrointestinal manifestations, produce hepatotoxicity and nephrotoxicity, and produce additive effects when used with opioid analgesics (Kumar *et al.* 2005). Many herbs, such as gingko, garlic, and ginseng, have potential anticoagulant effects. Such supplements should be avoided by patients who are thrombocytopenic, are taking medications with anticoagulant effects, or are in the peri-operative period (Weiger *et al.* 2002). The American Society of Anesthesiologists suggests that all herbal medications should be discontinued 2–3 weeks before an elective surgical procedure (Kaye *et al.* 2004).

## Counselling patients with cancer on herbal use

Physicians have an important role in educating their patients about herbs and helping them make informed decisions on the basis of critical appraisal of health claims. Physicians need to include queries about herbs and other supplements in medical histories and should ensure that the patient has undergone an appropriate conventional diagnostic assessment and been informed of all available conventional care options. In counselling patients about herbal products, it is important to be guided by the principle of 'do no harm'. Clinicians must be informed about the potential effects of herbal preparations and must be able to discuss this subject in a non-judgmental manner. They must tread the line between a sympathetic stance that might be interpreted as an endorsement of unproven therapies and categorical disapproval that would discourage the patient from revealing their use of herbal remedies.

Physicians should be aware that many patients will not reveal their use of herbal products unless asked. The discussion should be tailored to the individual, in an effort to convey professional views that they will understand and respect. In particular, patients should be informed that natural does not necessarily mean safe and that current labelling regulations in most countries do not ensure that the composition of the product contained in the bottle corresponds to what is on the label. They should also be informed that because current evidence is inadequate to predict which herbs may increase or diminish the effects of radiation or chemotherapy, it would be prudent to avoid combining these interventions until more information becomes available (Smith and Boon 1999; De Smet 2002; Weiger *et al.* 2002). Patients should be warned about misinformation on retail web sites, including sponsored sites. A review of 43 web sites that were assessed with regard to the quality and safety of the information presented about medicinal herbs, specifically in the field of cancer, revealed that most sites had low quality in a number of indicators including accuracy of information, revealing sources of information, biased presentation of information, or regularity of updates. Commercial sites had the most inaccurate or misleading information, emphasizing only the positive aspects of the herbs with little or no evidence. Seven percent of the sites discouraged the use of conventional medicine (Molassiotis and Xu 2004).

If a patient chooses to use herbal therapies, the physician should monitor the patient closely and remain alert for signs of adverse effects or interactions with conventional treatments.

## Popular herbs: Asian ginseng, Essiac, ginger, green tea, and mistletoe

### Asian ginseng

With the exception of one pilot study in which Asian ginseng appeared to improve fatigue in patients undergoing chemotherapy (Younus *et al.* 2003), no other trial helping to define the clinical utility of this herb in treating cancer or cancer-related symptoms was found. Asian ginseng has long been known for its preventive effects against a variety of cancers, including gastrointestinal, lung, and ovarian tumours, although it has no impact on prevention of cancers of the breast, thyroid gland, urinary bladder, or uterus (Boon and Wong 2004).

### Essiac

Essiac is a complex mixture of eight herbs and is usually consumed as a tea. Although some anti-cancer effects have been demonstrated at the laboratory level, it appears to be minimally effective clinically and published reports show mixed results. Essiac is one of the more popular herbal products used by Canadian cancer patients (Boon and Wong 2004). Prospective placebo-controlled randomized trials to gauge the efficacy of Essiac against cancer or to ameliorate symptoms are needed.

### Ginger

Two clinical trials (Boon and Wong 2004) and a recent meta-analysis (Chaiyakunaprur *et al.* 2006) showed ginger to be an effective intervention against chemotherapy-induced nausea and vomiting. Ginger could be seen as a reasonably effective adjunct with 5HT-3 drugs like ondansetron or granisetron, especially in patients who may not be able to take prochlorperazine or metoclopramide due to their side effects or when nausea and vomiting are refractory to the use of such drugs.

## Green tea

In four different clinical trials, green tea was found to have minimal or no effect against solid tumours, including lung cancer and hormone-refractory prostate cancer (Boon and Wong 2004; Choan *et al.* 2005; Laurie *et al.* 2005). Many studies have reported a preventive effect of green tea for a variety of cancers, including breast, gastrointestinal, lung, ovarian, prostatic, and urinary system tumours, as summarized in a recent review (Boon and Wong 2004). A significant dose–response relationship was evident in multiple trials. However, a number of other trials have reported either no benefit or increased risk of such tumours with green tea consumption. Thus, the literature does not support a clearly established preventive role of green tea.

## Mistletoe

Three retrospective case analyses and two prospective randomized trials have reported a potential survival advantage for patients treated with mistletoe (Boon and Wong 2004; Augustin *et al.* 2005). However, five other trials, in a variety of oncology settings, failed to show any significant improvement in disease-free or overall survival (Bar-Sela and Haim 2004; Boon and Wong 2004). A reduction in adverse reactions has been seen when mistletoe is used with cytotoxic therapies (Boon and Wong 2004). Mistletoe has been used as a loco-regional treatment to treat superficial bladder cancer and malignant pleural effusions with reasonable benefit (Boon and Wong 2004; Elsasser-Beile *et al.* 2005). Perhaps careful selection of tumour type and stage of the disease in properly designed randomized trials will help to establish the role played by this herb.

Details on the results reported by research studies on these five herbs are shown in Table 16.1.

### Case study

Mrs SJ, who is 48 years of age, has stage IV breast cancer with bone and liver metastases. She is presently receiving chemotherapy, which includes doxorubicin and cyclophosphamide. She had a recent deep-vein thrombosis and is taking daily warfarin. During a recent visit to her medical oncologist, he inquires as part of the medication history taking as to whether she is using any NHPs such as herbal medicines or other supplements. Mrs SJ says that she is not but that she has been experiencing mild nausea and thought some powdered ginger

**Table 16.1** Evidence base for Asian ginseng, Essiac, ginger, green tea, and mistletoe

| Herb | Cancer type | Study type | N | Dosage (including duration) | Outcome measure | Comments | Reference |
|---|---|---|---|---|---|---|---|
| Asian ginseng | Various solid tumours | Double-blind placebo-controlled pilot study | 20 | 250 mg Korean ginseng orally three times a day | Fatigue and overall quality of life improved with ginseng | | Younus et al. (2003) |
| Essiac | Various tumours | Consumer survey | 1162 | Variable | Symptom improvement in fatigue, appetite, nausea, pain etc. | Possibility of placebo effect is high | Boon and Wong (2004) |
| Ginger | Leukaemia | Double-blind, randomized pair, placebo-controlled design | 41 | Encapsulated ginger given over a 2-day period (details on dose not provided) | Significantly decreased severity and duration of nausea; no significant differences in terms of severity, frequency, and duration of vomiting or comfort level | | Boon and Wong (2004) |
| Ginger | Not specified | Randomized, prospective, crossover, double-blind study | NA | T1: Powdered ginger root; T2: Metoclopramide; T3: Ondansetron | Complete control of nausea was achieved in 62% (T1), 58% (T2), and 86% (T3) of patients; complete control of vomiting was achieved in 68% (T1), 64% (T2), and 86% (T3) of patients | Cyclophosphamide with other chemotherapy agents; patients had experienced at least two episodes of vomiting in the previous cycle | Boon and Wong (2004) |

| Herb | Cancer | Study type | N | Dose | Result | Notes | Reference |
|---|---|---|---|---|---|---|---|
| Green tea | Advanced lung cancer | Phase I trial | 17 | GTE[1] 0.5–3 g/m²/day | Maximum tolerated dose was 3 g/m²/day | Dose-limiting toxicity included diarrhea, nausea, and hypertension; no objective responses seen | Laurie et al. (2005) |
| Green tea | Solid tumours | Open-label, uncontrolled | 49 | Oral GTE at doses 0.5–5.05 g/m²/day or 1.0–2.2 g/m² three times a day with water for 4 weeks to 6 months | No significant responses observed | | Boon and Wong (2004) |
| Green tea | Hormone refractory prostate cancer | Open-label, uncontrolled | 19 | GTE 250 mg twice daily | Minimal clinical benefit found | Majority of patients had progressive disease within the first 4 months. | Choan et al. (2005) |
| Green tea | Hormone refractory prostate cancer | Open-label, uncontrolled | 42 | Green tea 6 g/day in 6 divided doses | Tumour response, defined as a decline ≥ in the baseline PSA value, was occurred in a single patient | All patients were asymptomatic and had progressive PSA elevation with hormone therapy | Boon and Wong (2004) |
| Mistletoe | Superficial urinary bladder cancer | Open-label, uncontrolled study Phase I/II | 30 | 50 ml of mistletoe lectin/week x6, concentration between 10 and 5000 ng/ml | Prevention of recurrence was similar to adjuvant BCG | No local or systemic side effects | Elsasser-Beile et al. (2005) |

**Table 16.1** (cont.)

| Herb | Cancer type | Study type | N | Dosage (including duration) | Outcome measure | Comments | Reference |
|---|---|---|---|---|---|---|---|
| Mistletoe | Bladder | Randomized, non-blinded, controlled study | 477 | Eurixor®-ML-1 standardized mistletoe preparation | Adjusted hazard ratio for DFS was 0.959 (95% CI = 0.725–1.268) | | Boon and Wong (2004) |
| Mistletoe | Malignant melanoma | Multi-centre, epidemiological, cohort study | 686 | Standardized *Viscum album* L.; subcutaneous injections 2–3 times weekly | Survival benefit in stage II–III; HR=0.41, p=0.002 | | Augustin et al. (2005) |
| Mistletoe | Malignant melanoma | Randomized, controlled, Phase III adjuvant trial, non-blinded | 407 | Iscador M® escalated from 0.01 to 1.0 mg/ml, over 2 weeks; after 3 days without treatment, injections were resumed for 14 doses (28 days) of 20 mg/ml followed by 7 days of no treatment | Disease-free interval: hazard ratio estimates for the comparison of Iscador M® versus control = 1.32 (0.93, 1.87); overall survival rate = 1.21 (0.84, 1.75) | High-risk patients with tumour thickness > 3 mm and or positive lymph nodes | Boon and Wong (2004) |
| Mistletoe | Metastatic colorectal | Phase II trial; open-label, non-randomized | 25 | 0.15–15 mg/day; subcutaneous injections | No objective tumour response seen | | Bar-Sela and Haim (2004) |

| | | | | | |
|---|---|---|---|---|---|
| Mistletoe | Colorectal | Randomized, controlled study | 64 | Isorel® mistletoe extract | Significantly better median survival and a better cumulative proportion survival rate in patients treated with mistletoe | 40 patients Stage Dukes C and 24 patients Stage D, mistletoe given as add on to surgery and chemotherapy | Boon and Wong (2004) |
| Mistletoe | Colon, rectum, stomach, breast, small cell or non-small cell lung cancer | a: Prospective, matched-pair cohort study, b: Randomized matched pairs | a: 792; b: 112 | Iscador® mistletoe extract | a: Survival time of patients treated with Iscador (4.23 years) was ~ 40% longer than in the control groups (3.05 years; $p < 0.001$) b: Statistically significantly longer survival time was reported in the Iscador group compared with the control group | | Boon and Wong (2004) |
| Mistletoe | Breast, ovarian and non-small cell lung | Multi-centre, randomized, open-label | 233 | Helixor® A at escalating doses ranging 1–200mg (standardized mistletoe extract) or lentinan (control) during chemotherapy according to treatment protocol for at least 4 months | Improved quality of life ($P < 0.05$) with fewer side effects | Conjunction with conventional cancer treatments | Boon and Wong (2004) |

**Table 16.1** (cont.)

| Herb | Cancer type | Study type | N | Dosage (including duration) | Outcome measure | Comments | Reference |
|------|-------------|------------|---|------------------------------|------------------|----------|-----------|
| Mistletoe | Breast | Retrospective cohort analysis with parallel groups | 1248 | EURIXOR™ (lectin-standardized mistletoe extract) | Reduction of adverse reactions and longer mean time to relapse in mistletoe group. No significant differences in survival or metastasis-free interval | Patients undergoing cytotoxic treatment | Boon and Wong (2004) |
| Mistletoe | Hepato-cellular carcinoma | Open-label, non-randomized, phase II study | 23 | 2 ampoules of Viscum fraxini-2 (aqueous solution containing 15 mg extract of mistletoe herb 20 mg from ash tree, diluted in dinatriummono-hydrogen phosphate, ascorbic add, and water) administered subcutaneously once weekly, for a median duration of 17 weeks, | 3 (13.1%) patients achieved complete response, 2 (8.1%) achieved a partial response, 9 (39.1%) had progressive disease, 9 (31.9%) patients did not have evaluation of response due to early death; median overall survival time for all patients was 5 months (range:2–38 | | Boon and Wong (2004) |

| Mistletoe | Malignant pleural effusions | Open-label, non-randomized, uncontrolled clinical study | 18 | Intrapleural treatment with Helixor® | ...months); median progression-free survival for all patients was 2 months (range: 1–38 months) Overall response rate for pleurodesis was 72% | Boon and Wong (2004) |
|---|---|---|---|---|---|---|
| | | | | | range 3–152 weeks | |
| Mistletoe | Renal adenocarcinoma | Open-label, uncontrolled, Phase II study | 14 | Subcutaneous injections of Iscador® every second day in escalating doses over 3 weeks followed by maintenance therapy: 20, 30, and 50 mg/ml on respective days | No response was demonstrated. Histologically verified renal adenocarcinoma stage IV and clearly measurable lung metastases | Boon and Wong (2004) |
| Mistletoe | Pancreatic | Retrospective case series | 320 | Subcutaneous Iscador® mistletoe extract injection, 2 or 3 times weekly, doses ranging 0.1 to 30 mg | Median survival time better or at least in the upper ranges, compared with stage reported in the literature. Patients' characteristics showed a prognostically unfavourable predominance of advanced stages of the disease | Boon and Wong (2004) |

[1] GTE, Green tea extract

might help. She has also contemplated taking Asian ginseng to help stimulate her immune system and help with her fatigue. She asks her medical oncologist for his opinion on these herbs. He shares with her his two main concerns. First, he is aware that both ginger and Asian ginseng have potential anticoagulation effects. He fears that if she were to take these herbs, he will be unable to maintain a therapeutic range of anticoagulation and that there may be an increased risk of bleeding. Second, with Asian ginseng having antioxidant properties, he is also concerned that there may be an alteration in the effects of chemotherapy, as both the chemotherapeutic agents used on her may rely on free radical and reactive oxygen species to mediate their cytotoxic effects. He is also aware that both the chemotherapeutic agents used on her are metabolized by the CYP450 enzymes and that Asian ginseng is believed to inhibit CYP1 activity. He worries that this may also negatively affect drug levels of her chemotherapeutic agents. He acknowledges that early studies suggest that Asian ginseng might help with fatigue and that the ginger might help with nausea but given the possibility of negative effects in her particular case recommends against their use at this time. Mrs SJ is receptive to her medical oncologist's concerns and chooses to abstain from taking these NHPs.

# References

Augustin, M., Bock, P. R. *et al.* 2005, Safety and efficacy of the long-term adjuvant treatment of primary intermediate- to high-risk malignant melanoma (UICC/AJCC stage II and III) with a standardized fermented European mistletoe (Viscum album L.) extract. Results from a multicenter, comparative, epidemiological cohort study in Germany and Switzerland. *Arzneimittelforschung*, vol. **5**, pp. 38–49.

Bar-Sela, G. & Haim, N. 2004, Abnoba-viscum (mistletoe extract) in metastatic colorectal carcinoma resistant to 5-flourouracil and leucovorin-based chemotherapy, *Medical Oncology*, vol. **21**, pp. 251–5.

Benzi, G. & Ceci, A. 1997, Herbal medicines in European regulation, *Pharmacological Research*, vol. **35**, pp. 355–62.

Block, K., Gyllenhaal, C. & Mead, M. 2004, Safety and efficacy of herbal sedatives in cancer care, *Integrative Cancer Therapies*, vol. **3**, pp. 128–48.

Boon, H. & Wong, J. 2004, Botanical medicine and cancer: a review of the safety and efficacy, *Expert Opinion in Pharmacotherapy*, vol. **5**, pp. 2485–501.

Boon, H., Stewart, M., Kennard, M. A. *et al.* 2000, Use of complementary/alternative medicine by breast cancer survivors in Ontario: prevalence and perceptions, *Journal of Clinical Oncology*, vol. **18**, pp. 2515–21.

Chaiyakunaprur, N., Kitikannakorn, N., LeepraKobboon, K. *et al.* 2006, The efficacy of ginger for the prevention of postoperative nausea and vomiting: a meta-analysis, *American Journal of Obstetrics and Gynaecology*, vol. **194**, pp. 95–9.

Choan, E., Segal, R., Jonker, D. *et al.* 2005, A prospective clinical trial of green tea for hormone refractory prostate cancer: an evaluation of the complementary/alternative therapy approach, *Urological Oncology*, vol. **23**, pp. 108–13.

De Smet, P. 2002, Herbal remedies, *New England Journal of Medicine*, vol. **347**, pp. 2046–56.

Elsasser-Beile, U., Leiber, C., Wetterauer, U. *et al.* 2005, Adjuvant intravesical treatment with a standardized mistletoe extract to prevent recurrence of superficial urinary bladder cancer, *Anticancer Research*, vol. 25, no. 6C, 4733–6.

Kaye, A., Kucera, I. & Sabar, R. 2004, Perioperative anesthesia clinical considerations of alternative medicines, *Anesthesiology Clinics of North America*, vol. 22, pp. 125–39.

Kivisto, K., Kroemer, H. & Eichelbaum, M. 1995, The role of human cytochrome P450 enzymes in the metabolism of anticancer agents: Implications for drug interactions, *British Journal of Clinical Pharmacoogy*, vol. 40, pp. 523–30.

Kruijtzer, C., Beijnen, H. & Schellens, J. 2002, Improvement of oral drug treatment by temporary inhibition of drug transporters and/or cytochrome P450 in the gastrointestinal tract and liver: an overview, *Oncologist*, vol. 7, pp. 516–30.

Kumar, N., Allen, K. & Bell, H. 2005, Perioperative herbal supplement use in cancer patients: potential implications and recommendations for presurgical screening, *Cancer Control*, vol. 12, 149–57.

Laurie, S. A., Miller, V. A., Grant, S. C., Kris M. G. & Ng, K. K. 2005, Phase I study of green tea extract in patients with advanced lung cancer, *Cancer Chemotheapy and Pharmacology*, vol. 55, pp. 33–8.

McCutcheon, A. R. & Beatty, D. 2000, Herb Quality. In *Herbs: Everyday reference for health professionals*, (ed) F. Chandler, Canadian Pharmacists Association, Nepean, Ontario. pp. 25–33.

Molassiotis, A. & Xu, M. 2004, Quality and safety issues of web-based information systems about herbal medicines in the treatment of cancer, *Complementary Therapies in Medicine*, vol. 12, pp. 217–27.

Porter, E. 1997, Herbalism. In *A History of Healing*, (ed) E. Porter, Marlow and Company, New York. pp. 68–93.

Smith, M. & Boon, H. 1999, Counseling cancer patients about herbal medicine, *Patient Education and Counseling*, vol. 38, pp. 109–20.

Sparreboom, A., Cox, M., Acharye, M. & Figg, W. 2004, Herbal remedies in the United States: potential adverse interactions with anticancer agents, *Journal of Clinical Oncology*, vol. 22, pp. 2489–503.

Weiger, W. A., Smith, M., Boon, H., Richardson, M. A., Kaptchuk, T. J. & Eisenberg, D. M. 2002, Advising patients who seek complementary and alternative medical therapies in cancer, *Annals of Internal Medicine*, vol. 137, pp. 889–903.

Younus, J., Collins, A., Wang, X. *et al.* 2003, A double blind placebo controlled pilot study to evaluate the effect of ginseng on fatigue and quality of life in adult chemo-naïve cancer patients. Abstract #2947, *Proceedings of ASCO* (22), p. 733.

Chapter 17

# Homeopathy

Elizabeth A Thompson

## Summary

The homeopathic approach is influenced by a complex view of health and disease and is underpinned by the philosophy that each person is unique and may benefit from an individualized prescription. Remedies can be derived from animal, mineral, or plant sources. Consultation style is patient led, symptom or problem orientated, and benefits from sensitive listening skills and an innate curiosity on the part of the prescriber to discover the nature of the problem. This process can resemble a palliative care approach—collecting information on patient concerns and symptoms and taking into consideration the social, spiritual, and psychological aspects that contribute to the human response to suffering.

## History and philosophy of homeopathy

It was Samuel Hahnemann (1755–1843), a German physician and scientist, who first began to uncover the central tenets of homeopathic philosophy. Whereas Descartes had reduced the human body to a machine, Hahnemann believed that *the vital force* animates and regulates the human form and directs growth, healing, and repair. He postulated that the homeopathic remedy acted through this vital force stimulating a healing response.

Hahnemann also developed *the law of similars*. He drew out patterns of symptoms in relationship to homeopathic medicines, in a process called Proving. The first proving (*pruefung*, meaning a trial of a substance) used *Chinchona*, the Peruvian Yew bark, known for its beneficial action in malaria and from which quinine was eventually derived. When given to a healthy person, this produced a pattern of symptoms similar to those found in the malaria sufferer. Hahnemann went on to build up a catalogue of these symptom pictures with a variety of substances including *Belladonna* (deadly nightshade) and *Arsenicum album*. These symptom pictures particular to a medicine could be matched to symptoms in a sick person. Having discovered that medicines given in this way could be curative in acute diseases, he stated the fundamental law of similars, 'let like be treated with like'. Some psychotherapeutic techniques might be said to share this homeopathic approach: focusing, clarifying, and reflecting back the same story with the hope of stimulating a healing response. Examples of conventional drugs that create the symptoms they are used to treat, thereby demonstrating the homeopathic principle, include amphetamine, which induces hyperactivity and is used in hyperactivity disorder; aspirin, which has hyperthermia as a side effect and is used in fever; and chemotherapy, which can induce malignant change and is used to treat malignancy. Provings are done to this present day as there are countless plant, mineral, and animal substances whose symptom pictures could be ascertained.

A third central concept is the *minimum dose*. Hahnemann sought the smallest amount of a substance that could be given to avoid side effects and would yet bring about a healing response. To his surprise, at some of the lower doses, the curative action of certain preparations seemed to be stronger, particularly when shaken vigorously (*succussion*). Hahnemann used the term *potentization* to describe the preparation of a homeopathic medicine using serial dilution and succussion.

To summarize three central tenets of homeopathic philosophy:

- Human beings have a regulating mechanism responsible for growth, repair, homeostasis, and healing through which the homeopathic remedy acts
- Matching the symptom picture so that the medicine is homeopathic to the symptoms is stated within the law of similars. Provings give information about the homeopathic symptom picture
- The minimum dose—homeopathic medicines are ultra-dilute and highly succussed

## Preparation of homeopathic medicines

After initial trituration (grinding) of the substance, the mixture is subject to a process of dilution and succussion (serial agitation against a hard surface), known as potentization. This leads to different strengths of medicines, for example, 6C is of low potency, whereas 200C is stronger. It is counter-intuitive to imagine that a substance can become more potent after being rendered more dilute. However, research suggests these highly succussed dilutions can be active and that it may be the succussion rather than the dilution that is the key to activating the solution.

## Laboratory research

One theory that has been put forward with ultra-molecular dilutions is that water may carry information, just like ferrous oxide can be a carrier for sound.

Beneveniste, who described this idea, supported research that demonstrated a biological action of an ultra-molecular dilution of anti-IgE (Davenas *et al.* 1988). His department was subsequently closed down but 13 years later, similar results were reported in a multi-centre European study (Belon *et al.* 1999). The research teams confirmed that high dilutions of histamine do indeed inhibit anti–IgE-induced basophil degranulation. It has been hypothesized that water could act as a template for the molecule and that since the dilution needed to be accompanied by vigorous shaking or succussion, transmission of the biological information could be related to the molecular organization of water. One study demonstrated thermo-luminescence patterns of ultra-molecular (15c) dilutions of lithium and sodium chloride (Rey Louis 2003). Thermally stimulated luminescence has proved to be an interesting tool to study the structure of solids, mainly crystals. The luminescence or glow that emerges from a crystal is characteristic of that crystal and depends on the trapping of electron pairs within the structure during activation at low energy using radiant energy such as X-rays or gamma rays. The homeopathic dilutions of lithium and sodium chloride were made in heavy water (deuterium instead of hydrogen) and when tested, the thermo-luminescence spectrum of the ultra-molecular dilutions resembles that of dilutions actually containing molecules of the substances. The team was surprised by these results and concluded that the structural state of a solution made in heavy water can be modified by the addition of selected solutes such as lithium and sodium chloride. This modification remains even when the initial molecules have disappeared and the effect is the same at different irradiation doses and for different radiant sources. As a working hypothesis, they believe that this phenomenon results from a marked structural change in the hydrogen bond network initiated at the onset by the presence of the dissolved ions and maintained in the course of dilution due to the succussion process. Clearly, more research is needed to investigate what appears to be a radical conceptual leap in our understanding of solutions.

## Clinical research

While basic science struggles to identify a mechanism of action for homeopathy, clinical research is accumulating evidence, with more than 100 randomized controlled trials being carried out. However, research specific to the cancer setting is very much in its infancy.

The role of a powerful consultation effect has been put forward as a key factor initiating the positive changes associated with the administration of the homeopathic remedy. However, clinical responses to ultra-molecular preparations have been shown in randomized placebo-controlled trials and the majority of meta-analyses have shown more than placebo effects. A recent but oddly designed meta-analysis based around the implausibility of homeopathy used only nine trials for the final analysis and did not show more than a placebo response (Shang *et al.* 2005). It was used to signal the 'end of homeopathy', reflecting the strong feelings often evoked within the medical establishment when discussing this topic. This was again reflected in a letter to *The Times* written by 13 eminent physicians, encouraging primary care trusts around the UK to stop all funding of homeopathy, citing a lack of evidence for efficacy (Baum *et al.* 2006).

The emerging evidence base in the cancer setting has strands from case histories, observational studies, and randomized trials with a recent systematic review (Milazzo *et al.* 2006). One case history in the palliative care setting describes the integration of homeopathy to enhance symptom control, whereas observational studies and randomized trials have shown improvements in anxiety and depression and a range of physical symptoms including fatigue, hot flushes, chemotherapy-induced stomatitis, and side effects of radiotherapy (Clover 1995; Balzarini *et al.* 2000; Oberbaum *et al.* 2001; Thompson and Reilly 2003; Jacobs *et al.* 2005). The systematic review of the efficacy of homeopathy in cancer yielded positive results in five of the six trials. Clearly, it is too early in the evolving evidence base for any one study as yet to signal the 'end of homeopathy'.

## Homeopathy in clinical practice

Different strategies are used to guide the choice of a homeopathic medicine, for example, *Arnica* can be used in a first aid setting for soft tissue damage with bruising and is recommended around the time of surgery for women undergoing mastectomy. This is referred to as a *local prescription* rather than an individualized one. Another approach called *isopathy* uses the causative agent as a remedy for the condition, for example, homeopathic house dust mite for patients with allergy, and has been extensively employed in homeopathic trials. It does not demonstrate the principle of similarity of a symptom complex and would be regarded as a weaker stimulus than a homeopathic remedy matched to the individual. *Complex remedies*, particularly common in Europe, combine several remedies put together for a particular clinical indication and are often sold over the counter. However, the gold standard of homeopathic care is the individualized prescription, also known as *classical homeopathy*, in which the totality of symptoms is taken into account. Classical prescribers would avoid polypharmacy as found in complex prescribing, as they would feel the similia principle in its pure form does not apply. *Tautopathy* involves prescribing a drug in potency, for example, homeopathic 5FU for a patient who has experienced difficult side effects from this drug. It is important to be able to distinguish between these different modes of prescribing of drugs when interpreting research data. In classical homeopathy, the individualizing process is central. In any trial that tests individualized prescriptions, the type of prescription cannot be controlled for and neither can the consultation process, which in itself is thought to be therapeutic and a vehicle for non-specific or placebo effects (Blackstone 1993). Complex or isopathic trials avoid consultation effects, as the same treatment is given to each patient for the same clinical condition.

The homeopathic community debates which approach is most effective but most prescribers agree that the closely matched similar using the totality of the symptom picture is the ideal approach and when accurate, leads to the strongest stimulus (Blackstone 1993). This is why case studies suggest that one remedy may not produce any response whereas another, which fits the symptom pattern more closely, may be followed by dramatic improvement in key symptoms as well as non-specific improvements in psychological adjustment. This comes back to the concept of homeopathacity and the similia principle, which drives case taking to greater degrees of detail. As homeopaths become more experienced, they are able to bring coherence to the developing symptom picture and identify remedies more accurately. A recent conceptual framework known as 'the levels', devised by an internationally acclaimed homeopath, has brought a greater understanding of how we build the totality of this symptom picture. We move down from the level of symptoms into the level of emotion, further into the level of delusion or how the individual views their world, and finally to the level of the vital sensation, the energetic disturbance that we are trying to match (Sankaran 2004). At the same time, we use the gestures and the language of the patient to identify the natural kingdom—plant, mineral, or animal—which is most likely to suit their inner nature.

- Level 1: Diagnosis—Some systems of medicine would not move beyond the diagnosis in managing the problem. 'You have a lump, it is cancer let's cut it out'
- Level 2: Symptoms—Modern medicine deals with symptoms as a means to confirm the diagnosis and surgery or a drug is usually prescribed
- Level 3: Emotions—Holistic approaches in general will begin to take into account how feelings influence any illness
- Level 4: Delusion or world view—The deeper energetic or vital disturbance colours everything including how the person perceives the world
- Level 5: Vital sensation—Reflects the deeper energetic disturbance that we are trying to identify and reflects the body's 'intelligence'

## Case 1

This lady has been referred by her oncologist with bilateral lymphoedema and very difficult chest wall pain since bilateral mastectomy 10 months previously. (Levels 1 and 2).

*Tell me about the lymphoedema.* 'I get this tightening here (*she makes a gesture tightening her arms around her chest*) and under the arms. It feels very tight, like there is a ring around my arm. It can feel hot and swollen as if it is joined together.' (Levels 4 and 5)

*Tell me more about the tightness.* 'It is really tight (*she clenches her fist*) I can only sleep on my back now and I have to move in stages. I can do a bit of housework but it is if something is stuck. It does stop me doing a number of things.'

*This is good, just describe more.* 'It is like a band, as if someone has put a vice on me (*she clenches her fist again*), as if there is a ring or tourniquet on the arm, as if everything is tightening and it won't release. I want to undo what is happening. I want release.'

*What is the opposite of this feeling?* 'Then I am opened back up again. I feel light and my body is working. It is like the arteries in my body are tight and vice like.'

This lady was able to move easily from her diagnosis to symptoms and to the deeper vital sensation making identification of the remedy she needed relatively straightforward. The vital sensation is that of the cactus family, with tightness and shrinking and the opposite light and open. I prescribed *Cereus bonplandii* as a liquid.

*Follow-up 6 weeks later:* 'I feel newborn, so much more confident. I took it daily for five days and then continued Monday, Wednesday, Friday, but it began to get tight again so I stopped and there was a marked improvement. I feel as if I am really getting back to two years ago, before this all happened.' She has a classical aggravation of her symptoms followed by a marked amelioration.

*Reviewed 5 months later:* 'Energy levels are brilliant. I was so tight as if in a vice as if my skin would burst and I felt so drained. Now I can do everything with my arms. It was tightening and tightening like a vice but now it is as if someone has undone the screws there is release. I feel better than before I had the diagnosis of cancer.'

## Case 2

A gentleman with locally recurrent chondrosarcoma complaining of stiff aching in left hip (Levels 1 and 2).

*Describe the pain?* 'Squeezing, tight, cramped, freedom in life is restricted.'

*Tell me more about restricting?* 'It's restricting my flowing movement. Tennis is my sport— it is like dancing—your whole body moves as one—blue skies open up.' (Levels 4 and 5)

*The opposite?* 'Heavy cloud—your body shrinks and closes up.'

*Tell me about shrunk and closed up?* 'Shrinks, body is smaller, the energy is depleting, deflating, like a balloon—a deflated tyre.' (Level 5—language of the vital sensation).

*The opposite?* 'Bouncing around vibrant—a balloon at bursting point, liberating full of joy. No weight of expectation. I am big, floating, six feet tall.'

*Dreams?* 'There are people but no relation, no connection to them. I cannot connect with this woman in my dream. An incredible bond, a powerful deep connection, the ultimate connection. I feel lonely, empty. Like when I am tensed up, lost empty and cold, flat, devoid of energy.' (Level 3 the language of emotion and level 4 delusion—I am alone in the world.)

*The opposite?* 'I am almost not there. I am floating and rarefied, out of body, no impediments. I am there as well but I have merged. It is stunningly beautiful.'

Here we see the vital sensation of a gas and in this case *Hydrogen* is the remedy. It went through a proving in 1991 and has the themes of having no sense of structure, spaced out and floating with a great sense of connection or a great sense of disconnection and isolation. This case shows that it was only with the newer method of encouraging patients to trust their bodies' inner wisdom and use the physical symptoms to guide us to the vital sensation that a good remedy such as *Hydrogen* was revealed.

Six months after starting *Hydrogen* : 'I am doing very well—my scan is clear and my energy is good. It is very strong and consistent and my back feels secure. There is solidity and support. I feel I have got myself a solid foundation. I feel strong, solid, feel I am appreciated for what I am doing in my work, emotionally sustained. The remedy is an amazing support—it is steadfast.

## Tools to assist the homeopath in finding a good match for the individual

- *The Repertory*: This book lists thousands of symptoms arranged in sections according to their anatomical site of origin. Alongside each symptom is recorded all the remedies that include this symptom in their picture, for example, Chest; CANCER; Mammae; injuries, after (2): con., hyper

- *Materia Medica*: This complements the repertory by listing remedies along with their characteristic symptoms. Information from toxicology, provings, and clinical experience are collected together to create a comprehensive picture for each remedy

Both these tools are now available as computerized software.

## Problems encountered using the homeopathic approach

Much of homeopathic philosophy is based around the ideal of health and the expectation of full recovery. What is not yet clear is what outcome can be hoped for using the homeopathic approach in the cancer setting. Cancer sufferers are a vulnerable group of people and fostering unrealistic expectations may engender denial or false hopes of recovery. Offering homeopathy as another approach to symptom control, rather than suggesting that remedies can have an impact on the disease itself, is more realistic.

There are no known toxic effects of homeopathy. However, there can be reactions suggestive of a shift within the self-regulating mechanism thought to orchestrate the body. If the method of developing symptom pictures is to give the medicine to healthy volunteers, then giving repeated doses could lead to the symptoms of the remedy appearing over time. These are called new or proving symptoms, which are fairly unusual because in most cases just a few doses of the medicine are given. A worsening of existing symptoms followed by an improvement is called a homeopathic aggravation. In a recent audit of 116 patients in routine outpatient practice, one-third of patients described aggravations and new symptoms and five patients regarded the aggravation as adverse (Thompson *et al.* 2004). Homeopathic aggravations can lead to confusion if there are other causes for an apparent deterioration. The homeopathic medicine should be stopped and the aggravation should settle quickly. The remedy can then be restarted at a lesser frequency of administration. Regular reviews are essential.

Finally, it has been suggested that homeopathic remedies that are based on the principle of tautopathy, for example, homeopathic vincristine given concurrently with vincristine as a conventional chemotherapy agent, may interfere with the action of the conventional drug. Research has shown that mesangial cells in the rat's kidney can be protected from cadmium poisoning by pretreating with homeopathic cadmium. Whether homeopathic remedies might affect excretion rates of a poison is unclear and more research is needed as the overall effect may be a positive one to reduce chemotherapy side effects without affecting cancer cell killing.

## Homeopathy as part of the National Health Service

Great Britain has five homeopathic hospitals (London, Bristol, Liverpool, Tunbridge Wells, and Glasgow); all run entirely within the National Health Service and having active audit and research programmes. For doctors and other healthcare workers, there is both full-time and part-time training in homeopathy, leading up to the Primary Healthcare Examination. Doctors can take studies further and sit the Membership of the Faculty of Homeopathy. This faculty, set up by Act of Parliament in 1950, is at present developing a basic training through to specialist qualification.

## Conclusion

The homeopathic approach is a complex intervention, which is increasingly popular with patients. The individualizing process of choosing the remedy may in itself be therapeutic and research design should acknowledge this complexity. Qualitative research may illuminate the therapeutic nature of the doctor–patient relationship that develops through this consultation process. Clinical efficacy can be explored through pragmatic randomized trials, a design that appears acceptable in other areas of healthcare. The gold standard of the placebo-controlled randomized trial needs particular thought as regards both design and interpretation of results. The evidence base for homeopathy in the cancer setting is still in its infancy but a systematic review suggests that patients with cancer have benefited from homeopathic interventions, specifically for chemotherapy-induced stomatitis, radiodermatitis, and symptoms of oestrogen withdrawal in breast cancer survivors. More research is urgently needed to provide patients with choices in their care but in the meantime, the approach appears safe and inexpensive with minimal side effects and levels of satisfaction are high (Spence *et al.* 2005).

## References

Balzarini, A., Felisi, E., Martini, A. & de Conno, F. 2000, Efficacy of homeopathic treatment of skin reactions during radiotherapy for breast cancer: a randomised, double-blind clinical trial, *British Homeopathic Journal*, vol. **89**, no. 1, pp. 8–12.

Baum, M. B. C. B. G. *et al.* Full letter: doctors' campaign against alternative therapies. The Times Online, available at http://www.timesonline.co.uk/article/0,,8122-2191985,00.html (accessed August 1, 2006).

Belon, P., Cumps, J., Ennis, M. *et al.* 1999, Inhibition of human basophil degranulation by successive histamine dilutions: results of a European multi-centre trial, *Inflammation Research*, vol. **48**, Suppl 1, pp. 17–8.

Blackstone, V. 1993, Single or multiple prescribing - a debate, *British Homeopathic Journal*, vol. **82**, pp. 37–52.

Clover, A. 1995, Complementary cancer therapy: a pilot study of patients, therapies and quality of life, *Complementary Therapies in Medicine*, vol. **3**, pp. 129–33.

Davenas, E., Beauvais, F., Amara, J. *et al.* 1988, Human basophil degranulation triggered by very dilute antiserum against IgE *Nature*, vol. **333**, no. 6176, pp. 816–8.

Jacobs, J., Herman, P., Heron, K., Olsen, S. & Vaughters, L. 2005, Homeopathy for menopausal symptoms in breast cancer survivors: a preliminary randomized controlled trial, *Journal of Alternative and Complementary Medicine*, vol. **11**, no. 1, pp. 21–7.

Milazzo, S., Russell, N. & Ernst, E. 2006, Efficacy of homeopathic therapy in cancer treatment, *European Journal of Cancer*, vol. **42**, pp. 282–9.

Oberbaum, M., Yaniv, I., Ben Gal, Y. *et al.* 2001, A randomized, controlled clinical trial of the homeopathic medication TRAUMEEL S in the treatment of chemotherapy-induced stomatitis in children undergoing stem cell transplantation, *Cancer*, vol. **92**, no. 3, pp. 684–90.

Rey, L. 2003, Thermoluminescence of ultra-high dilutions of lithium chloride and sodium chloride, *Physica A*, vol. **323**, pp. 67–74.

Sankaran, R. 2004, *The Sensation of Homeopathy*. Homeopathic Medical Publishers, India.

Shang, A., Huwiler-Muntene, K., Nartey, L. *et al.* 2005, Are the clinical effects of homeopathy placebo effects? Comparative study of placebo-controlled trials of homeopathy and allopathy *Lancet*, vol. **366**, no. 9487, pp. 726–32.

Spence, D. S., Thompson, E. A. & Barron, S. J. 2005, Homeopathic treatment for chronic disease: a 6-year, university-hospital outpatient observational study, *Journal of Alternative and Complementary Medicine*, vol. **11**, no. 5, pp. 793–8.

Thompson, E. A. & Reilly, D. 2003, The homeopathic approach to the treatment of symptoms of oestrogen withdrawal in breast cancer patients. A prospective observational study, *Homeopathy*, vol. **92**, no. 3, pp. 131–4.

Thompson, E., Barron, S. & Spence, D. 2004, A preliminary audit investigating remedy reactions including adverse events in routine homeopathic practice, *Homeopathy*, vol. **93**, pp. 203–9.

Chapter 18

# Massage

Jacqui Stringer and Peter A Mackereth

## Summary

Massage involves the manipulation of soft tissues using a range of different techniques. The belief that a cancer diagnosis is a contra-indication to massage is largely unfounded, although adaptations of technique may be needed for individuals with cancer and it will not be appropriate in all cases. Published studies show that the benefits of massage in the cancer care setting include relief from anxiety, depression, pain, nausea, and insomnia. It may also improve measures of immune function. Guidelines for safe practice are given in this chapter.

## Introduction

Massage, in its many forms, is one of the most popular complementary therapies in cancer care. Historically and culturally, massage has been used since ancient times around the world. Hippocrates believed it to be an essential healing technique for all physicians to use (Grealish and Lomasney 2001). As an intervention, it can involve a range of strokes, rubbing, and palpation and pressure techniques to manipulate the soft tissues (skin, muscles, and tendons) of the body. Importantly, as a means of providing touch, it can communicate tenderness, comfort, and a sense of being present with another. Equally, if provided without care and sensitivity, it can be perceived as invasive, sometimes disturbing and even uncomfortable. It is important to ascertain potential benefits, risks, and costs to inform and enable service users and providers in considering this intervention. It is also important to consider individuals' receptivity to touch because some may associate physical contact with an earlier history of abuse, physical restraint, or invasive technical touch that caused pain (e.g. needle insertion, wound care, or medical investigation) or a sense of powerlessness and fear.

## Myths around massage in cancer care

There are a number of anxieties centred on the delivery of massage in the field of oncology. Two of the most common ones are considered here.

In the past, cancer was viewed as a contraindication to massage, the main reason being that rubbing soft tissues might 'spread cancer' through the lymphatic system. However, the forms of adapted massage used in this field are all very gentle; therefore, the level of pressure applied would be no greater than when patients rubbed themselves dry with a towel. It is noteworthy that any physical movement such as dressing, walking, and even breathing can encourage movement of fluids in the lymphatic system.

Another concern relates to the therapists' safety. Some therapists express concern about 'contaminating' themselves by exposure to chemotherapy and radiotherapy through physical contact with patients. However, there is no evidence to suggest that therapists are at risk from working with patients undergoing medical treatment for cancer.

These assumptions, and any others not based on evidence, need to be challenged formally, and investigated thoroughly so that the concerns of referrers, therapists, and patients can be addressed.

There may be situations when massage would be contra-indicated (as is the case in any area of practice), which is why it is critical that any therapist working with patients with cancer has a good understanding of the pathologies, treatments, and side effects of treatments patients are likely to encounter.

## Research work

Kahn (2001), a teacher of massage, recommends that training schools have an important role in transforming massage into a research-conscious profession.

There is now a growing body of research relating to massage for patients living with cancer. Cassileth and Vickers (2004) reported on a series of more than 1000 patients who received massage at the Sloan-Kettering Cancer Centre. Massage had an immediate and substantive beneficial effect by reducing symptoms of anxiety, depression, pain, and nausea. In outpatients, these benefits were still evident at least 48 hours later.

In another large study ($n = 230$) involving patients with cancer, Post-White et al. (2003) showed massage could improve ratings in several measures including anxiety and perception of pain.

From a slightly different perspective, patients with cancer have also been seen to be proactive in using complementary therapies, including massage, to both improve immune function and ease the side effects of cancer treatments.

Morris et al. (2000), in a postal survey enquiring about use of complementary therapies, received a total of 617 replies from the original 1935 questionnaires sent to a random selection of patients with cancer attending their centre. They discovered that 53% of these patients used massage.

The research group led by Professor Tiffany Field and Dr Maria Hernandez-Reif at the Touch Research Institutes in Miami, Florida, has shown that massage can improve various parameters of immune function, psychological state, and disease markers across a range of heath problems. In 34 women with early-stage (I and II) breast cancer, the team looked at mood, immune function, and levels of stress (Hernandez-Reif *et al.* 2004). Their results suggested massage to be beneficial in a number of ways, including significant reductions in anxiety and depression scores and enhancement of immune function through increase in numbers of natural killer (NK) cells in the massage group. Their data reflected a significant positive change in NK-cell numbers for the massage arm and a negative change for the control arm.

## Haematological cancers

The treatment of choice for patients with acute leukaemias is potentially curative and involves high-dose chemotherapy, which can paradoxically cause rapid deterioration in their physical condition so that they require nursing in protective isolation (Zittoun *et al.* 1999). These patients have traditionally been deemed too poorly for massage; consequently, there is a paucity of studies carried out in this environment. In spite of the difficulties, it has been shown that a safe service can be offered to this very needy group of patients (Stringer 2000; Stringer 2006) and there are studies that validate the concept of offering massage to patients with haematological malignancies and confirm its benefit to them.

In one randomized study ($n = 20$), parents in the experimental arm were trained to massage their children suffering from acute lymphoblastic leukaemia (Field *et al.* 2001). Both immediate and longer-term changes were measured in levels of anxiety and depression for parents and children. Additionally, variations in the children's white cell and neutrophil counts were monitored across the 30 days of treatment. Results from children in the massage arm were compared with those in a waiting-list control arm. A statistically significant reduction in depression scores over the study period was noted for parents performing the massage but not for those in the control group. The children who had been massaged also had a significantly greater number of white blood cells and neutrophils, which was not evident in children from the control group. Ahles *et al.* (1999) showed that in patients undergoing an autologous bone marrow transplant, massage led to reduction in diastolic blood pressure, nausea, distress, and anxiety. Smith *et al.* (2003) investigated outcomes following three different interventions for patients undergoing bone marrow transplantation. A number of perceived benefits from massage therapy were reported, including reduced scores for insomnia, anxiety, and depression.

## Assessment and contracting for massage

Careful assessment of all patients, particularly those undergoing active treatments or having altered immunity and/or haematological disorders, is essential in order to avoid massaging someone inappropriately. Such an assessment would include taking a history of their current condition, relevant past medical history, and documenting any side effects of medical treatment such as dry, flaky skin or erythematous reactions to radiation or drugs.

It is important to acknowledge that not all patients want to receive massage. Contracting to any form of physical contact is morally and ethically a hallmark of professional healthcare practice. All recipients of massage must be made to feel sufficiently empowered that they are comfortable in asking for the session to pause or stop (Mackereth 2000). Consent for touch is always an ongoing process and not dependent on signing a form to give permission, although it is appropriate for patients and therapists to give written consent to confirm their understanding of the mutual contract they are making.

## Adaptations

In private practice, massage for healthy people is typically delivered in the privacy of a therapy room, often with the client undressed, and for at least 40–60 minutes. Massage can be sensual, vigorous, deep, and powerful, leaving the body feeling profoundly relaxed, reinvigorated, maybe even achy for a few days. However, patients living with cancer may be fatigued, have lost weight, and be experiencing altered body image, making it difficult to receive touch or expose their bodies to others. It is therefore the responsibility of the therapist to consider adaptations, both in terms of techniques and length of treatment, for example:

- *Clothed work*: Working over a towel or blanket will soften the contact and provide warmth and modesty
- *Gentle techniques*: Use light touch and short moments of holding. This can involve gently releasing the hold with the patient's inspiration to encourage expansion of breath and a deeper letting go of the out-breath
- *Shorter treatments*: A maximum of 15–25 minutes, perhaps daily or twice weekly. Always contract for the length of the session and be mindful to take cues from the patient in case it needs to be drawn to an earlier close
- *Involve and teach carers*: This must be supervised and supported. Do not presume a family member, partner, or friend would feel comfortable with providing touch

- *4-Hands Holding* (Mackereth *et al.* 2000): This is paired working, where, for example, a partner or a second therapist contributes to the session by massaging the other hand or foot, or perhaps holds and strokes the patient's head

---

### Case 1

Joan, aged 75 years, with advanced lung cancer and dependant on oxygen therapy, was sleeping badly, exhausted, and anxious. The hospital's massage therapist attended her for 25-minute sessions prior to daily physiotherapy. After the first session, consisting of gentle massage to the neck, back, and feet, she was calmer and able to concentrate on working with the physiotherapist to make better use of her respiratory muscles and pattern of breathing. Gradually, over the week, her sleeping improved and she was strong enough to be discharged home. Joan died in her sleep a week later.

---

## Prophylactic abdominal massage

A distressing side effect of some chemotherapy drugs (for example, vincristine) and strong analgesics (for example, morphine), widely used for patients with cancer, is severe constipation. In extreme cases, this can result in bowel damage and the withholding of treatment. As a preventative measure, following prescription of such medication, patients can be trained in abdominal self-massage by a massage therapist (Mackereth *et al.* 2006). They would be encouraged to perform the routine from one to three times a day before food, their technique and progress being regularly monitored. Carers can also be taught so they can help the patient if desired.

## Providing massage for carers

Within the authors' practice area, a massage service to patients' relatives and visitors arose from requests from nursing staff to help support relatives, who are often tired, stressed, and anxious. Typically, they have placed their own lives on hold to be with their loved ones, who may be undergoing surgery, radiotherapy, and/or chemotherapy. Traditional massage has been performed in a prone or supine position, usually with some or all clothing removed and requiring at least 45 minutes for a full treatment.

At the Christie Hospital, Manchester, UK, a chair massage service was initiated in 2002 as a means of delivering treatment by the bedside, without asking recipients to undress and using an ergonomically designed chair (Fig. 18.1). This has proved to be very successful and has been well received. Evidence suggests that massage benefits carers in similar ways to patients; in a study by the Oregon Hospice Association and East-West College of Healing Arts (1998), 13 caregivers

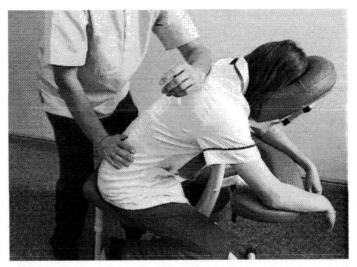

**Figure 18.1** Chair massage treatment.

were given an average of six massages. After the treatments, 85% reported reduction in emotional and physical stress levels, 77% reported reduction in physical pain, and 54% reported better sleep.

### Case 2

Rebecca, aged 52 years with breast cancer, was close to death. Her partner George and two young sons were in attendance. The nurses had asked the massage therapist to treat George, who had not slept for three nights and was agitated and uncommunicative with his sons. On arrival, the sons were standing by the window and George was leaning against the end of Rebecca's bed, watching her intensely. The therapist offered to treat him in a massage chair. After 25 minutes of massage, he was breathing deeply and even beginning to snore. The therapist finished by wrapping him in a large towel and encouraged him to sit by Rebecca. Without a word, he rested his head against Rebecca's side and closed his eyes. The two sons drew their chairs nearer and held him.

This service has grown in popularity and the practitioners have now developed a training course to share their experiences and expertise with massage therapists working in hospice and cancer care settings.

## Conclusion and recommendations

For the novice massage therapist, the idea of providing massage to a patient living with cancer may be daunting. Indeed, the advice would be not to provide treatment unless specific guidelines are developed and followed with clinical support and supervision given to ensure safe and skilled clinical practice. The following recommendations are made for best practice in providing massage within cancer care settings:

- ◆ Research and evaluation work is required to explore further the safety, efficacy, and specific outcomes of massage for people affected by cancer
- ◆ It is essential that consent for massage be a continuous and respected process, allowing a patient to say 'no' at any time during the session
- ◆ Myths need to be critically reviewed for validity
- ◆ Contraindications or cautions that would need skilful adaptation of the treatment, require assessment and evaluation on an individual patient basis
- ◆ Massage therapists require additional training to develop their knowledge of cancer and its treatments
- ◆ Continuing education and clinical supervision can help therapists to maintain and review their skills and knowledge
- ◆ There is a need to develop specialist massage practices, for example, lymphoedema management, that work with patients living with compromised immunity
- ◆ Carers can also benefit from massage, although this may need to be provided by the patient's bedside and without the need to undress

## References

Ahles, T. A., Tope, D. M., Pinkson, B. *et al.* 1999, Massage therapy for patients undergoing autologous bone marrow transplantation *Journal of Pain and Symptom Management*, vol. **18**, no. 3, pp. 157–63.

Cassileth, B. R. & Vickers, A. J. 2004, Massage therapy for symptom control: outcome study at a major cancer centre, *Journal of Pain and Symptom Management*, vol. **28**, no. 3, pp. 244–9.

Field, T. 2000, *Touch Therapy*. Harcourt Press, London.

Field, T. Cullen, C., Diego, M. *et al.* 2001, Leukaemia immune changes following massage therapy, *Journal of Bodywork and Movement Therapies*, vol. **5**, no. 4, pp. 271–4.

Grealish, L. & Lomasney, A. 2001, Massage. In *Complementary therapies in nursing and midwifery: from vision to practice*, (ed) P. McCabe, Ausmed Publications, Melbourne.

Hernandez-Reif, M., Ironson, G., Field, T. *et al.* 2004, Breast cancer patients have improved immune and neuroendocrine functions following massage therapy, *Journal of Psychosomatic Research*, vol. **57**, pp. 45–52.

Kahn, J. 2001, Research Matters. *Massage Magazine*. Issue 92 July/August.

Lively, B. T., Holiday-Goodman, M., Black, C. & Arondekar, B. 2002, Massage therapy for chemotherapy-induced emesis. In *Massage Therapy: the Evidence for Practice*, (eds) G. J. Rich, Harcourt Brace, London.

Mackereth, P. 2000, Tough places to be tender: contracting for happy or 'good enough' endings in therapeutic massage/bodywork? *Complementary Therapies in Nursing and Midwifery*, vol. 6, no. 3, pp. 111–5.

Mackereth, P., Campbell, G., Norman, M. *et al.* 2000, Introducing '4-Hands Holding': many hands make profound work, *Cahoots*, vol. 72, pp. 36–8.

Mackereth, P., Stringer, J. & Gray, D. 2006, Therapist as teacher. In *Massage & Bodywork: adapting therapies for cancer care*, (eds) P. Mackereth, & A. Carter, Elsevier, London.

Morris, K. T., Johnson, N., Homer, L. & Walts, D. 2000, A comparison of complementary therapy use between breast cancer patients and patients with other primary tumour sites, *American Journal of Surgery*, vol. 179, pp. 407–11.

Post-White, J., Kinney, M. E., Savik, M. S., Berntsen Gau, J., Wilcox, C. & Lerner, I. 2003, Therapeutic massage and healing touch improve symptoms in cancer, *Integrative Cancer Therapies*, vol. 2, no. 4, pp. 332–44.

Smith, M. C., Reeder, F., Daniel, L., Baramee, J. & Hagman, J. 2003, Outcomes of touch therapies during bone marrow transplant, *Alternative Therapies*, vol. 9, no. 1, pp. 40–9.

Stringer, J. 2000, Massage and aromatherapy on a leukaemia unit. *Complementary Therapies in Nursing & Midwifery*, vol. 6, pp. 72–6.

Stringer, J. 2006, Massage and essential oils in haemato-oncology. In *Massage & Bodywork: Adapting Therapies for Cancer Care*, (eds) P. Mackereth, & A, Carter, Elsevier, London.

Zittoun, R., Achard, S. & Ruszniewski, M. 1999, Assessment of quality of life during intensive chemotherapy or bone marrow transplantation, *Psycho-Oncology*, vol. 8, pp. 64–73.

## Website

Touch Research Institutes: http://www6.miami.edu/touch-research

Chapter 19

# Music therapy

Joanne V Loewy

## Summary

Music offers a unique and powerful channel of expression, independent of the use of words. Music therapy has been shown to have many benefits in the cancer care setting, including the reduction of anxiety, pain, and insomnia, and improvement in mood, well-being, and quality of life for both patients and caregivers. A detailed professional evaluation inclusive of a family assessment enables the formulation of a treatment plan that is catered to an individual plan of care. Techniques of music therapy used with this population can be complex. Three unique approaches—drumming, music visualization, and song review—are presented here.

## Introduction

Music therapy is the use of music to achieve emotional, physical, cognitive, and/or spiritual habilitation. Goal areas may include, but are not limited to, ego enhancement, improvement of motor skills, social/interpersonal development, cognitive development, self-awareness, and spiritual enhancement.

Music therapy provides a unique forum for discourse and expressive opportunity because, unlike verbal discourse, it does not require a person to construct meaning through an organized cognitive forum. Sounds and silences are a part of an on-going, live experience that exists temporally and viscerally for the human being from birth to death. How one adapts to the sound environment from moment to moment involves a host of experiences that include imposition, choice, adaptation, and organization. Such are the instances of structure, definition, composition, and human will that the music therapist is faced with when entering a human relationship.

This chapter will review the use of sounds, silences, clinical improvisation, song, and lullaby in the care of individuals facing cancer. Our understanding of musical and non-musical voyaging will provide a means of exploration from life to death along the human continuum, in the hope that the reader will gain knowledge about how silence, music, and music therapy may be an accessible modality. Sometimes this will be one of comfort, safety, and fortitude in disease and transition towards death. In other cases, this will impact the use of resistance and/or formation, hosting a province of wilful strength and vitality in sustaining life.

Music therapy as an accredited profession began in the mid-1900s. The Certification Board for Music Therapy is the only US organization to certify music therapists to practice music therapy nationally. Since 1986, it has been fully accredited by the National Commission for Certifying Agencies. More than 4000 music therapists have attained the MT-BC credential and now participate in a program of recertification designed to maintain or increase initial competence in the profession of music therapy (www.CBMT.org 2006). Music therapy may be included in the rehabilitative therapies section of the Health Care Financing Administration regulations (JAMA 1991) and music therapists are eligible for Medicare reimbursement.

The Louis and Lucille Armstrong Music Therapy Programs at Beth Israel Medical Center have been using music therapy in oncology and palliative care and also as a forum for nurses and other staff to release tension as they share feelings of loss, and address their own compassion fatigue, in a weekly session run by a music therapist. Creating community among the professional caregivers involved in the day-to-day difficulties in assisting patients with cancer and their families has been an important and unique aspect of our program (Stewart *et al.* in Dileo and Loewy 2005).

## Research on music therapy in cancer care

Gallagher *et al.* (2001) studied the effect of music therapy on 200 patients with advanced disease using visual analogue scales, the Happy/Sad Faces Assessment Tool, and a behaviour scale, with scores being recorded pre- and posttreatment. The results indicated that music therapy improved anxiety, body movement, facial expression, mood, pain, shortness of breath, and verbalizations. Sessions with family members were also evaluated and music therapy seemed to improve families' affectual range, as well as their mood and verbalizations. All improvements were statistically significant. Most patients and families showed a positive subjective and objective response to music therapy. Other studies on patients with cancer have shown improvement in mood and decrease in anxiety (Magill 2001; Cassileth *et al.* 2003), enhancement in quality and length of life (Hilliard 2003), assistance in relaxation in the ICU (Johnston and Rohaly-Davis 1996), and reduction of pain (Krout 2001; Magill 2001) as well as assisting in the general management of patients—both children and adult (Lane 1993).

A German study (Reinhardt 1999) carried out on patients suffering from chronic cancer pain found that a 30-minute lullaby-like, rhythmically dominated music with gradually decreasing tempo improved their ability to fall asleep. The intervention was a 14-day training in a relaxation therapy and the researchers recorded the following parameters: measurement of the continuous registration of heart rate and its comparison with musical beat on days 1 and 15; analysis of the degree of synchronization—coordination of systole and musical central time point; time of falling asleep; and the patient's subjective evaluation of the relaxation therapy and pain intensity. It was found that the music had a profound effect; the patients in the relaxation group showed an increasing synchronization and co-ordination of heart rate and musical beat. At a tempo of between 48 and 42 beats per minute, there occurred a very stable 2:3 synchronization pattern of heartbeats. Those patients reporting the best relaxation and analgesic effects showed the most synchronization. Music therapy also led to a decrease in consumption of analgesics.

## Assessment

The most important means of knowing how a person is coping with cancer or any progressive disease is through an evaluation. Adopting a comfortable but detailed means of learning about how a person comprehends the disease process, and also a way of sensing how various aspects of coping are or are not in place, is essential to how treatment is formulated.

Ideally, prior to developing a plan of care, the therapist will have had opportunities for individual music therapy assessment with the patient alone and then again with his/her family or significant other(s). A comparison of these two experiences will provide detailed information about coping mechanisms and reflect how the patient chooses to involve others or prefers to remain introspective during the process. There is an underlying trend in the literature and among those who work with the chronically ill and/or dying, that patients should not be alone and that family support is necessary. This may be an oversimplification of in fact what a clinician will develop within a plan of care in terms of social support.

This does not imply that those who work closely with patients should not try to understand and develop or strengthen a patient and family's means of support. Empathy for patients who are newly diagnosed, or have a progression of illness, or are terminally ill is critical. Yet, how and whom the patient desires to become involved in the care is a critical choice and too often assumptions are made about relationships based on a hurried gathering of data collected by admitting staff and reflected in the medical record. What a musical exchange may reflect in terms of intimacy and the delicate nuances of relationships within families might provide a host of information not yet either realized or fully understood through verbal discourse. I have worked with a handful of patients who desired to die alone and who did not have that opportunity at the time of death because of family needs and/or assumptions.

We are often so busy and invested in wanting to help and take care of patients that we do not spend enough time listening to their desires or discovering, through a therapeutic stance and process, the areas that are of most importance to them. As music is a metaphoric modality and may involve a listener as well as a performer, there are numerous vehicles for addressing a patient's deepest wishes and desires.

During an assessment, the music therapist provides a multitude of opportunities for the patient to express himself/herself spontaneously through instrumental play or song or through listening, whereby the patient can orchestrate the music he/she would like to have the therapist or family member play. The collaborations or avoidances of collaboration, style of music, elemental properties of the music, and historical and cultural contexts of selected music provide a host of important parameters that serve as a foundation for clinical treatment.

The silences are critical to the musical relationship. As silence provides an essential and special context for the sounds, a music therapist must be comfortable with space. Too often, therapists or those wanting to assist the patient fill in the exchange with words, offerings, questions, or even musical clutter. In working with patients who have a serious illness, it is gravely important to assess and be sensitive to the canvas of opportunity. The therapist frames the canvas but it is the patient who creates the art. If the frame or supportive music takes up too much space, the patient's intentions, desires, aesthetic preferences, and sense of creativity and playfulness becomes cramped and confined.

A tour of the room (Loewy 2000) provides the patient with opportunities to construct the sound environment. After the contact music and/or opening talk is finished, the therapist demonstrates the instruments and sounds available and suggests that the patient pay attention to how the sound affects the mood or how the patient is feeling in general.

The patient might request that the therapist play or he/she may select something to play. Musical interchanges might ensue. At some point, the favourite song or style of music may be revealed. There is usually a history connected to this preference. This is sacred information that is critical to treatment planning. The therapist takes careful musical notation and/or tapes the music if it is unfamiliar and the patient allows for such learning.

In the clinical context of music therapy, the relationship of the music between the therapist and patient and among the patient and family/friends or significant others is of utmost importance. The music has its unique dynamic inclusive of rhythm, dynamic, tempo, tone, melody, harmony, and timbre. These qualities and how they are combined in a relationship exist outside of the music in speech and body language but they also exist within the context of a musical relationship. The therapist takes careful note of this and may or may not choose to reflect upon it with the patient, depending on the patient status and the goals that have been overtly discussed or subtly referred to through the context of the musical or verbal relationship.

The music therapist must 'participate fully and authentically, feeling the raw emotion—the raw material—that shapes our sound' (Rykov 2001). In this way, the music is truly psychodynamic and human, which is of utmost importance in a medical musical psychotherapy context.

The Model of Integrative Medical Music Psychotherapy (Loewy and Scheiby 2001, unpublished) (Colour plate 5) provides a rationale for how music is specifically and holistically integrated within a medically driven treatment context. The musical parameters (colour coded) on the top correspond to the medical areas on the bottom. The mid-part of the model defines the psychospiritual conditions for the goals.

## The musical textures of treatment planning

A music therapy care plan is developed with structure and flexibility. The plan's course will depend largely on the level of illness the patient presents with and how much attention the patient desires to spend addressing the pending issues. Often, a diagnosis of cancer leads a person to become introspective and extremely private. This situation might call upon the therapist to be silent or to play music that is soft and slow, perhaps an improvisation with a minimal harmonic but an optimal thematic line.

Another patient may choose to ignore or deny the diagnosis. Music in this instance may be used as an escape or outlet whereby an improvisation leads towards a creative path of discovery. In this clinical context, the relationship may represent newness or a means of getting away from the heaviness or the trauma of what the cancer has brought about. This is honoured and respected. The patient steers the relationship and musical activity within the scope of spontaneity. Music in this case may bring about a feeling of resilience.

Yet another patient may ask the music therapist to simply play. It is not uncommon for a therapist to hear a patient with cancer say: 'Play … just play, anything, it doesn't matter what it is, just play'. This is a perfect opportunity for nurturance. The therapist must use his/her intuition, observation skills, and counter-transference to delineate what would be the most appropriate music or song to offer. There are many subtle factors that come into play during the decision making. What does the patient desire, but is afraid to ask? What is the patient's culture? What kind of taste does the patient present? Observing the clothing style, food in the room, or posters on the wall may indicate what is likely to create a feeling of comfort in this particular context.

Treatment is planned jointly between the patient and therapist, when possible and if appropriate. There is a plan at hand but it may shift, especially as the progression of illness changes. Therefore, the therapeutic relationship developed during the assessment and first few sessions is critical as it must endure any change in health status.

## Three common music therapy techniques and goals

### Drumming

Rhythm is the foremost vital sign among the human being and animal races. We are beings among an environment of rhythm in nature, as in the changing of seasons, the lightness and darkness of day and night. We count on time in our use of clocks, monitoring where we will spend each hour of the day. Beings are creatures of habit and repetition evokes in us a sense of fortitude and vitality. The heartbeat, or first audible sound within the womb, is the beat in which we regulate our breathing and pulse.

When a patient is medically examined, the heartbeat and rate is the first sound a physician might check to estimate a patient's health condition. Moreover, in day-to-day existence, we regulate our own moment-to-moment activities according to the clock. From second to second, day to day, month to month, year to year, season upon season, we sense the passage of time, in a rhythm we grow to understand more fully with each passing minute.

In working with rhythm in a conscious way, which is literally that which a drumming experience provides, we are able to experience a sense of mastery, groundedness, rootedness, and vitality when we are able to create rhythmic sounds. This rhythm elicits within us an ordered structure or may be created as part of a more free release-like experience. The rhythmic design we choose to set up resonates with our daily movement and functions. Whether we are waiting in our automobile for a red light to turn green or we are using an iPod on the stair master exercise machine to constantly maintain our impetus to move, we are always entraining to rhythm.

Drumming with or for patients with cancer can provide a sense of release and/or empowerment. This is the most basic way that I have used drumming in my work.

I have seen patients limp with fear come to terms with their inner power through drumming, perhaps a power they had forgotten they held. I have seen patients in the midst of ambivalence, or in purgatory, regain a sense of meaning and purpose because of releasing rhythms in synchrony as someone else followed, listened, and entrained with them.

Medically, drumming can be helpful to patients who are unconsciously with-holding. I have used drumming to help patients who were constipated move their bowels and/or bladder. I remember a 50-year-old male patient who had bowel cancer. He had a catheter for voiding. After 30 min of drumming, he told me that he wanted to urinate. For the first time in 3 months, he was able to urinate naturally, without a catheter.

We understand the concept of releasing as a technique in pain management. When a person stubs his/her toe, there is a sudden, sharp pain. Yelling, for even a quick second, may provide a moment of release. Patients with cancer are often faced with discomfort, pain, and/or nausea. Drumming can provide a means of pain release. At the same time, it is a means of being heard and resonance may occur as another individual plays in synchrony with the person who is in pain. This can be powerful and the pain may decrease or even subside.

If we look at other cultures where painful rituals are a part of transformation, we might see body piercing or fire walking. Within these rituals are drumming sounds. When one drums with full intention and concentrated energy, the pain is not noticed and the pain cycle or response might be shut down completely. Many clinicians believe that pain and music responses travel along the same neural pathways. Since rhythm is an instinctual response, drumming is an important option of control and release.

## Music visualization

Although drumming may provide a sense of structure or a means of release, not every patient will feel comfortable using the drum as a means of treat-ment. Drums offer a forum for bringing energy outside of the body. Many choose to hold their energy inward and become increasingly private and introspective during their illness. Music visualization may provide a unique modality of healing.

The therapist may suggest a variety of genres by simply playing for the patient and watching the response. This may work particularly well for patients who are in a coma. For the patient who can express the music of choice, the therapist can attend to the breathing rate of the patient and entrain the meter of the music to the patient's respiration. This may evoke a relaxation response.

An extension of such an activity would be to suggest that the patient select and image a place of comfort and safety. The music played for the patient may provide a unique means of relaxation. This might address fear that has kept someone from sleeping or prevented them from trusting that when they go to sleep, they will die. Music can be heard as one sleeps and can soothe, much like a lullaby sung by the mother or the father of a patient when he/she was a young child.

Music may be useful in creating a remembrance of an infant stage of development. This may assist in offering a sense of completion in the life cycle. Many patients have requested lullabies or songs of kin (Loewy *et al.* 2005) that were used in their childhood. The request to die with such a song and family surrounding or enveloping the bedside is not uncommon.

## Song view and review

Whether cancer has brought one towards a transition at the end stage of life or towards gaining a sense of new vitality in order to live more fully, the use of song and song review may provide a powerful means of contextualizing or framing significant periods, people, moments, and circumstances for therapeutic intervention.

At a most basic level, a person's selection of song may be reflective of important information. Singing favourite songs for, and/or with, patients and families may by itself be therapeutic. The astute music therapist will keep track of the songs and carefully view the thread-line theme potential of the selections, not only through lyric interpretation but also within the dynamic, key, style, and timbre and in the way that the song is sung. If a patient does not sing, it would be important to ask how he/she desires the song to be sung—slow, fast, high, low, and on what instrument as accompaniment, or *a cappella*. The song used in therapy has an amorphous life of its own.

While working further with song, whether dying or simply hospitalized for a treatment, creating a song autobiography can be a useful endeavour that provides patients with clarity. The songs can be sewn together from particular periods of significance or be patient-composed based on particular people, time periods, or places. Patients have used songs to remember and then in singing their autobiography reflected on aspects of their life that they desire to change for the future or finish before dying. The scope of desire delved upon in years of clinical sessions has provided a vast range of expression and intention.

Patients have written songs for family members, using the autobiography model to relive and express musical snapshots of precious moments or used humour to express anger, or love songs from weddings to one-word instrumental verses about the need for forgiveness. Whatever the intention or desire, songs and autobiographies provide a means and a context for expression, reflection, reconstitution, and possible closure, whether ultimately as in death, or alternatively in burying a particular issue so one can feel more able to live the next stages more fully.

## Conclusion

This chapter has provided a theoretical rationale for the use of music therapy as applied in the clinical context of treating patients with cancer. The central aspects of treatment are applied only upon careful in-depth music therapy assessment and evaluation. The plan of care is drawn from the music therapy evaluation in tandem with the treatment team's input and consideration.

The three types of music therapy applications described are not meant to imply that these are the only ones available but are taken from the contextual review of many applications within the author's years of experience. It is hoped that the reader will find these applications helpful and when and if possible a consultation with the team be made, ensuring that the patient will be held by a sense of collaboration and unified experiences in life and in death.

## References

Cassileth, B., Vickers, A. & Magill, L. 2003, Music therapy for mood disturbance for hospitalization for autologous stem cell transplant: a randomized controlled trial, *Cancer*, vol. **98**, no. 12, pp. 2723–9.

Gallagher, L., Huston, M., Nelson, K., Walsh, D. & Steele, A. 2001, Supportive care in cancer, *Music Therapy in Palliative Care*, vol. **9**, no. 3, pp. 151–61.

Hilliard, R. 2003, The effects of music therapy on the quality and length of life of people diagnosed with terminal cancer, *Journal of Music Therapy*, vol. **40**, pp. 113–37.

Johnston, K. & Rohaly-Davis, J. 1996, An introduction to music therapy: helping the oncology patient in the ICU, *Critical Care Nursing Quarterly*, vol. **18**, pp. 54–60.

*Journal of the American Medical Association*, vol. **26**, no. 10, September 11, 1991.

Krout, R. E. 2001, The effects of single-session music therapy interventions on the observed and self-reported levels of pain control, physical comfort, and relaxation of hospice patients, *American Journal of Hospice and Palliative Care*, vol. **18**, pp. 383–90.

Lane, D. 1993, Music therapy: gaining an edge in oncology management, *Journal of Oncology Management*, Jan/Feb, pp. 42–6.

Loewy, J. 2000, Music psychotherapy assessment. *Music Therapy Perspectives*. AMTA, Fall, 2000.

Loewy, J., Hallan, C., Friedman, E. & Martinez, C. 2005, Sleep/sedation in children undergoing EEG testing: a comparison of chloral hydrate and music therapy, *Journal of Perianesthesia Nursing*, vol. **20**, no. 5, pp. 323–31.

Magill, L. 2001, The use of music therapy to address the suffering in advanced cancer pain, *Journal of Palliative Care*, vol. **17**, pp. 166–72.

Reinhardt, U. 1999, Investigation into synchronization of heart rate and music rhythm in a relaxation therapy in patients with cancer pain, *Forschende Komplementaermedizin*, vol. **6**, no. 3, pp. 135–41.

Rykov, M. H. 2001, Facing the music: speculations on the dark side of our moon, *Journal of Palliative Care*, vol. **17**, no. 3, pp. 188–92.

Stewart, K., Silberman, J., Loewy, J. *et al.* 2005, The role of music therapy in care for the caregivers of the terminally ill. In *Music Therapy at End of Life*, (eds) C. Dileo, & J. Loewy, Jeffrey Books, Cherry Hill, NJ.

## Chapter 20

# Nutrition

Elizabeth Butler

## Summary

There is strong evidence that dietary factors are important in carcinogenesis and that many cases of cancer could be prevented by improvements in diet. The influence of nutritional status on the length and/or quality of life for those already diagnosed with cancer has not yet been thoroughly studied. However, a growing body of research literature suggests that good nutritional support for people with a history of cancer can have numerous benefits: preventing the malnutrition that is so common in this population, preventing the spread or recurrence of cancer, preventing other degenerative diseases, alleviating symptoms of cancer and side effects of treatment, enhancing emotional well-being, and enabling patients to take more active control over their health.

## Introduction

It is estimated that between 20 and 40% of people with cancer die of malnutrition, rather than the direct effects of the disease (National Cancer Institute 2005). This statistic alone justifies the special attention that needs to be paid to the nutritional requirements of patients with cancer. The high level of malnutrition in this population is due to increased demands for particular nutrients, and nutritional status being undermined by the disease and its treatment.

The benefit of nutritional support for cancer patients with acute nutritional needs is well recognized. Research results in this and other fields of hospital medicine have firmly established that well-nourished patients respond better to treatments and suffer fewer complications. Far less attention has been paid to the potential benefits of nutritional support in addressing the long-term health needs of cancer survivors, although this is starting to change.

Research indicates that when cancer survivors are not provided with information and support on how to live well with their disease, they often seek ways to help themselves. One area they frequently choose to investigate is nutrition and they will be rewarded with an abundance of literature that may either gratify and reassure or, considering the amount and contradictory nature of the information, will overwhelm and confuse.

Many experts believe that those living with cancer should be routinely offered nutritional advice and support from health professionals. After all, the links between diet and cancer are known to be strong, with the World Health Organisation estimating that dietary factors account for 30% of cancers and the World Cancer Research Fund saying that 30–40% of cancers could be prevented with dietary changes. However, the vast majority of research on nutrition and cancer has focused on prevention of the disease and less is known about the effects of diet in those already diagnosed. Of course, prevention is still an important issue for cancer survivors—prevention of further disease spread, cancer recurrence, and secondary cancer development.

Apart from any possible influence on the cancer process, nutritional support could benefit cancer survivors in other ways. This population is at increased risk of developing other degenerative conditions such as cardiovascular disease, osteoporosis, and diabetes. Many of these diseases have clear links with diet and can be prevented, or their effects minimized, by healthy lifestyle choices.

Another important way in which dietary changes could support the physical health of cancer survivors is through positive effects on mental and emotional states. Evidence shows that patients who actively engage in their treatment and recovery process gain a sense of control that leads to a reduction in stress. One area where patients can truly engage is their diet.

This chapter will explore dietary components that may support or undermine the health of those living with cancer. Details of a supportive diet are given, along with nutritional recommendations to alleviate some common symptoms. Some of the research studies quoted are concerned with cancer prevention but also have probable relevance to people living with cancer.

## Dietary factors as anti-cancer agents

The idea that foods can influence the development of cancer has existed for hundreds of years. As the evidence for links between diet and cancer has grown stronger in recent decades, scientists have investigated the effects of individual foods on cancer development and progression and a selection has emerged as having particularly potent anti-cancer activity.

Plant foods score most highly in this area, important examples being green tea, garlic, tomatoes, mushrooms such as maitake and shiitake, soya foods, the spice turmeric, and berry fruits. Certain animal products also offer anti-cancer benefits, in particular the oily fish.

These foods, or the nutrients within them, possess a range of activities that inhibit certain aspects of the cancer process. Almost all possess powerful antioxidant activity, some directly regulate the immune system, others possess anti-angiogenic activity, some influence the endocrine system and others display anti-inflammatory effects. Many dietary components are active in all these ways and more.

Table 20.1 provides an overview of some foods with anti-cancer properties. Many others also show promise but research is still in the preliminary stages. It is important to note that the components currently deemed to be the primary anti-cancer components may later be found to form just part of the picture as scientists continue to investigate the complex interactions of the array of chemicals within our food.

**Table 20.1** The anti-cancer components present in certain foods

| Food | Primary anti-cancer components | Anti-cancer actions | Research |
|---|---|---|---|
| Green tea | Epigallocatechin and epigallocatechin gallate | Antioxidant, induce apoptosis, anti-angiogenic, has positive influence on cellular communication | Studies have shown that green tea provides protection against cancer and also indicate that several cups per day can impact on disease recurrence (Inoue et al. 2001) |
| Berries e.g., blackberries, blueberries, strawberries | Anthocyanins, anthocyanidins, and proanthocyanidins | Antioxidant, anti-angiogenic, actions that undermine tumour invasion and metastasis | Laboratory and animal studies have identified cancer-suppressive effects of chemicals found in various berries |
| Tomatoes | Lycopene | Antioxidant, improves cellular communication and signalling, up-regulates the detoxification enzymes | In supplement form has been shown to influence progression of existing disease in men with prostate cancer (Kucuk et al. 2002) |
| Garlic | Allyl sulphur compounds | Antimicrobial, antioxidant, induces apoptosis, up-regulates the detoxification enzymes | Garlic extract has been shown to prevent decline in natural killer cells in people with advanced cancer (Ishikawa et al. 2006) |

(continued)

**Table 20.1** (*cont.*)

| Food | Primary anti-cancer components | Anti-cancer actions | Research |
|---|---|---|---|
| Turmeric | Curcumin | Antioxidant, anti-inflammatory, anti-angiogenic and anti-metastatic | Trials testing the effects of curcumin in patients with cancer are underway currently (Sharma *et al.* 2004) |
| Medicinal mushrooms e.g., Maitake, Shiitake, and *Coriolus* versicolor | Beta glucans | Immune stimulation and modulation | In certain Eastern countries, a lot of research has been conducted and extracts of mushrooms such as maitake, shiitake, and *Coriolus* versicolor are licensed medicines. In the Western countries, scientific interest is growing. |
| Soya | Isoflavones– genistein, diadzein | Phytoestrogen– anti-oestrogen effect, antioxidant, anti-angiogenic, re-differentiation | Epidemiological evidence suggests a possible connection between soya in the diet and reduced cancer risk. |
| Oily fish | Omega-3 essential fatty acids | Anti-inflammatory, immune modulation | Some evidence suggests that supplements of omega-3 fatty acids can have a positive influence on the health of those with cancer (Nakamura *et al.* 2005) |

# Dietary factors as cancer-promoting agents

Dietary factors that appear to play a role in promoting cancer include naturally occurring compounds such as saturated fats, alcohol, refined carbohydrates, sugar, and caffeine; chemicals formed during the manufacturing or cooking process such as acrylamide, trans fats, and heterocyclic amines; and additives such as sodium nitrite and aspartame. The foods most likely to contain these compounds are processed and refined foods; sugary or fatty items such as chips, biscuits, confectionary, and red meat; tea and coffee; and alcoholic drinks.

Certain of these foods are not inherently unhealthy, particularly the natural ones such as red meat. Their potential negative effect is influenced by factors such as the quantity consumed and the quality both of that particular food and the rest of the diet.

Food components directly affect the biochemistry of the body and so can influence the cancer process in a variety of ways. Dietary fats can have a significant impact on immune function, their metabolic by-products directly affecting the inflammatory response. Recent research has confirmed the idea that a low level of inflammation is part of the disease profile in cancer (Balkwill and Mantovani 2001). Fats with the potential to promote an inflammatory response in the body include the saturated fats, the omega-6 essential fatty acids, and the trans fats. High levels of dietary saturated fats are not recommended for people with cancer and the level of omega-6 fats should ideally not exceed the optimal omega 6:omega 3 ratio, which is believed to be 4:1 (Hardman 2004). Trans fats are best excluded from the diet completely.

Refined carbohydrates and caffeine may also affect the immune system by influencing the inflammatory response. Both these food components can lead to a steep rise in blood glucose, which can lead to insulin resistance, a factor associated with low-level inflammation and linked to increased cancer risk (Giovannucci 2003; Chen 2006). The few studies that have considered the direct impact of refined carbohydrates on cancer development and progression tend to show a positive association (Bravi *et al.* 2007).

Alcoholic drinks are often high in sugar and it may be partly for this reason that they have the effect of increasing cancer risk. Alcohol probably also has direct carcinogenic effects and although these are yet to be fully defined, they probably include the genotoxic effect of acetaldehyde, which is the main metabolite of ethanol.

A number of other food components have known, or suspected, direct carcinogenic activity. These include acrylamide, a compound produced in starchy foods cooked at high temperatures; the heterocyclic amines produced when meats are browned; sodium nitrite, a preservative added to processed meats; and aspartame, a sweetening agent. Excluding these substances from the diet is advisable for those with a history of cancer.

## Diet and cancer survivorship studies

In recent years, a few studies have considered the effects of whole diets on the health of those with cancer, measuring various outcomes including length of survival, disease progression, development of secondary cancers, and quality of life.

Ornish *et al.* (2005) reported a randomized controlled trial which found that a vegan diet, nutritional supplements, stress management techniques, and exercise had a positive influence on the progression of early-stage prostate cancer in men. Of course, the diet was only one aspect of this intervention, making it impossible to determine its precise effect. Similar results using a plant-based diet with minimal animal products were found in a small case-series study (Saxe *et al.* 2001). The positive results of these studies should encourage researchers to conduct larger trials.

## A diet to support the health of the cancer survivor

Some would consider that it is too early to offer dietary advice to those with cancer because the research about survivorship is still preliminary. However, healthy eating guidelines for disease prevention are well established and the prevention of further tumours or the spread of existing ones is obviously important for people with cancer, as is the prevention of other chronic conditions. The basis for the dietary programme detailed in this chapter is a well-recognized, common-sense approach to healthy eating, developed and adapted to meet the specific needs of the cancer survivor.

The diet that appears most suitable for the person living with cancer is based on fresh, natural ingredients, ideally organic, and prepared in the home. This means a move away from factory-processed convenience foods, which can be a big change for some individuals or families. Inspiring cookbooks are essential in facilitating this change along with much guidance and support from those qualified to provide it.

Evidence abounds when it comes to the virtues of a plant-based diet for general health (Trichopoulou *et al.* 2003). Therefore, although this diet contains small amounts of unprocessed animal products, the majority of foods are derived from plants. Fruit and vegetables feature prominently due to their powerful anti-cancer properties and ideally, a person with cancer would consume 8–10 portions daily, although digestive problems may inhibit this initially. For many, this is a significant leap and so simple ideas on boosting fruit and vegetable intake are required, examples being the use of home-made juices and smoothies, crudites and dips, or fresh fruit as snacks, and salad starters before a main meal.

Other important plant foods are the whole grains, pulses, nuts, and seeds. A wide selection of each would be ideal and the more unusual varieties such as the highly nutritious grains quinoa and millet would be encouraged. Such foods are good sources of fibre and essential vitamins and minerals. Many are cancer-protective for other reasons, such as their phytoestrogen content. Some can be sprouted to enhance nutritional value.

Nuts and seeds also provide the body with essential fats, as do the oily fish. While nuts and seeds are generally richer in the omega-6 essential fats, the oily fish contain more of the omega-3. Much research has focused on the health effects of individual dietary fats, but as discussed earlier, it is the overall balance that is most important in determining effects on health. A diet providing a healthy balance of fats will contain minimal fatty meats and dairy products (these contain saturated fats), be free from fatty processed foods such as cakes, biscuits, chips, and crisps (these contain the trans fats), and will feature oily fish regularly along with nuts and seeds. Vegetable oils can be used in moderation, but only olive or coconut oil are recommended for cooking, their chemical structure allowing for less damage when heated. Although coconut oil contains saturated fats, not all saturated fats affect health in the same way and those abundant in coconuts (the medium-chain saturated fats) appear to have anti-inflammatory activity (Ohta *et al.* 2003).

People with cancer are also advised to avoid foods high in salt or refined sugar. Many people love sweet foods and are heartened to realize that puddings, cakes, and biscuits made with healthy ingredients and sweetened using dry fruits can form part of their diet.

This section would be incomplete without discussion of dairy products and the soya bean products often promoted as healthy alternatives to dairy. In recent years, the idea that milk and milk products could undermine the health of those with cancer and even encourage the disease to spread has been highlighted in certain popular books. The main reason is the presence of natural growth factors in milk. Laboratory and animal studies indicate that these growth factors can stimulate cancer cell proliferation (Foulstone *et al.* 2005). These data are insufficient for making dietary recommendations and there have not yet been any studies directly addressing the question of whether dairy is suitable for cancer survivors. Looking to the cancer prevention data, research indicates that dairy may slightly increase the risk for some cancers (breast, ovary, and prostate), while may decrease it for others (colorectal).

The suitability of dairy may also be questioned due to the presence of saturated fats, although lower fat products solve this problem, and lactose intolerance. Many people treated for cancer experience digestive upsets including diarrhoea. The milk sugar lactose can exacerbate this problem and in such cases, dairy foods are best avoided.

Overall, the question of whether dairy foods are advisable has to be addressed on an individual basis. Despite the concern over bone health for those on a dairy-free diet, it is perfectly possible to obtain sufficient calcium and other bone-supporting nutrients from a good range of other healthy foods, in particular green leafy vegetables, nuts and seeds, dry fruit, oily fish (especially those with edible bones), pulses, whole grains, and olives.

Many people who choose to avoid dairy switch to products made from soya beans. Despite the positive research around soya isoflavones, soya foods do have a negative side. The soya bean contains antinutritional factors, such as trypsin inhibitors, which can interfere with nutrient digestion and absorption. In countries where soya forms part of the staple diet, it is usually processed so that levels of the antinutrients are reduced. In the West, this may not occur to the same extent. If people choose to eat soya foods, those produced in a more traditional manner such as tofu, miso, and tempeh are recommended. Those who want to avoid both dairy and soya milk can use rice, oat, or nut milk.

## Nutritional supplements to support the health of the cancer survivor

Increased nutritional requirements as a result of metabolic changes and the high demands of recovery, together with the common disruption to oral intake, food digestion, and nutrient absorption, mean that even a healthy diet may not meet the nutritional needs of a patient with cancer. Loss of appetite, particularly around the time of treatment or towards the terminal stage, further reduces the chances of all the necessary nutrition being obtained from food.

For those with cancer, nutritional supplements can therefore be very useful or even essential as a back up to the diet. Pre-prepared high-energy supplementary drinks are sometimes prescribed to patients who would not receive adequate calories otherwise. The problem is that these drinks are processed and contain large amounts of refined sugars. Many people also find them unpalatable. Ideas for tasty, home-made, high-energy drinks are given in the following section.

Most nutritional supplements taken by patients with cancer are unprescribed and include vitamins, minerals, and phytonutrients, singly or in combination. They may have been recommended by a health practitioner, such as a nutritional therapist, or may have been chosen by the patients themselves. Supplements that can be particularly beneficial in support of a good diet include a multivitamin and mineral, an omega-3 essential fatty acid product, and an antioxidant product, ideally one containing a wide range of antioxidant vitamins, minerals, and phytonutrients.

Some concern has been expressed by health professionals regarding the use of nutritional supplements alongside primary cancer treatment. In particular, there has been speculation that antioxidant supplements may interfere with chemotherapy or radiotherapy. There is also some research evidence that antioxidants may benefit people having these treatments by reducing their toxicity (Nicolson 2005). Although there is not enough evidence to draw firm conclusions, current knowledge suggests it is advisable for patients with cancer to stop taking antioxidants close to the time of treatment. Supplements can be resumed between treatments to encourage regeneration and healing.

## Nutritional support for cancer signs and symptoms

Nutritional support has something to offer to all people with cancer, whether they are in the earliest stages of disease or receiving palliative care. Ensuring that the body is supplied with optimal levels of the essential nutrients will support general health, leading to stronger defence mechanisms and greater healing capacity. Specific foods and nutritional supplements can also be used for the management of specific symptoms.

Digestive problems are common and should be treated as a priority issue. Even a perfect diet will not improve nutritional status significantly if digestive and absorptive capacity is impaired. Damage to the gut lining and disruption to the balance of gut microflora are often at the root of digestive problems. Use of the amino acid–like compound glutamine and the herbs marshmallow, slippery elm, and *Aloe vera* to soothe and heal the gut wall along with some pre- and probiotics to rebalance the gut microflora can result in dramatic improvements in digestion. Digestive enzymes can also be useful.

Fatigue is another very common complaint. There is no easy solution to this problem and the body may simply need extra rest at this time. However, nutritional support will help ensure that deficiencies of particular nutrients are not exacerbating the problem.

Freshly prepared juices provide nutrients in a form that can be rapidly and efficiently absorbed (McEligot *et al.* 1999) and are fantastic for supporting the health of the weakened patient. Ideally, juices should be vegetable based, with just a little fruit to sweeten, thereby minimizing any rise in blood sugar. Vegetables and fruits that are ideal for consumption as juices include carrots, beetroot, dark salad leaves, apples, and fennel. Herbs and spices can also be included in juices for their specific healing properties. Different foods have specific beneficial effects, as illustrated in Table 20.2.

Many people experience changes in weight at some point following a cancer diagnosis. Either weight gain or weight loss may occur depending on the cancer site and both have a negative impact on prognosis (Chlebowski *et al.* 2002; Argiles 2005). The healthy eating programme previously described can be very useful in assisting those who need to lose weight. The healthy eating programme is also appropriate for those who need to gain weight; however, the details discussed in the subsequent text need to be borne in mind.

The view that calories, regardless of their source, are the priority for underweight patients with cancer is still commonly held by mainstream health professionals although research shows the ineffectiveness of calorie loading as a stand-alone treatment in helping patients to gain and maintain weight (Brown 2002). One reason for this is that the metabolic changes occurring in

**Table 20.2** Healing properties of fruit and vegetables recommended for juicing

| | |
|---|---|
| **Apple**<br>Rich in pectin, a substance that can help lower cholesterol levels. Apple juice is a good source of a range of nutrients and it mixes well with most other juices | **Lettuce**<br>Has a natural calming and sedative effect Is very cooling and thirst quenching. Dark lettuce leaves contain higher levels of nutrients |
| **Beetroot**<br>Rich source of iron and other blood-building minerals. Powerful liver cleanser but too much consumption at once can cause nausea | **Orange**<br>Rich source of vitamin C and bioflavanoids, both powerful antioxidants. Juice the nutrient-rich pith as well as the flesh if possible |
| **Broccoli**<br>Contains compounds known as indoles that support liver detoxification and in particular enhance the breakdown of oestrogens | **Parsley**<br>Rich source of chlorophyll and other blood-building nutrients. Acts as a blood cleanser |
| **Cabbage**<br>Like broccoli contains the indole compounds. Contains compounds that soothe and heal the digestive tract | **Pear**<br>A good juice for promoting detoxification and elimination. Soft pears will clog the juicer, hard ones should be used |
| **Carrot**<br>Rich source of carotenoids that possess powerful antioxidant activity. A good cleansing juice that mixes well with other juices | **Pepper**<br>Rich source of antioxidant compounds including vitamin C. Green peppers have a strong taste and work best mixed with other juices |
| **Celery**<br>A natural diuretic helps to remove excess fluid from the body. Has a strong flavour and is best combined with other juices | **Pineapple**<br>Contains powerful anti-inflammatory agents. Aids digestion |
| **Cranberry**<br>Contains natural antibacterial compounds, useful for urinary tract infections. A rich source of powerful antioxidant phytonutrients | **Radish**<br>Helps to clear mucus from the system and is good for respiratory problems. Acts as a blood cleanser |
| **Cucumber**<br>Is very cooling and thirst quenching. A mild diuretic | **Tomato**<br>Rich in antioxidant, anti-tumour compounds such as carotene and lycopene |
| **Ginger**<br>Adds a warming element to a juice. Possesses cardiotonic, anti-inflammatory and antibacterial properties. A natural anti-sickness remedy | **Watercress**<br>Rich source of chlorophyll and other blood-building nutrients. Rich source of antioxidant compounds. Peppery taste can be strong, mix with other juices. |

cancer that trigger weight loss are driven by the action of cytokines as part of the inflammatory response. Foods high in animal saturated fats, trans fats, and sugars have a pro-inflammatory effect in the body. Foods that are high in calories but at the same time supportive to the body include coconuts, avocados, oily fish, nuts, and seeds. These foods can be used to encourage weight gain. Fruit smoothies are a great way of providing someone who is losing weight with extra calories and nutrients in an easy-to-digest form. An example of a high-calorie smoothie recipe, based on one developed by Penny Brohn Cancer Care, is given below. It can be adapted to suit individual tastes and for variety. Any type of soft or dry fruit can replace the blueberries and banana, silken tofu can be added to increase the protein content, and coconut milk can be added to increase calories. Medium-chain triglycerides are abundant in coconuts and are particularly beneficial for those losing weight as they are readily digested and absorbed and readily provide energy.

## Recipe for blueberry and avocado smoothie

| | |
|---|---|
| Sesame seeds | 1 tsp |
| Whole almonds | 1 tsp |
| Hemp seeds (shelled) | 1 tsp |
| One medium banana | 110 g |
| Plain yoghurt (dairy or soya) | 100 ml |
| Half a large avocado | 75 g |
| Blueberries | 100 g |
| Rice milk | 125 ml |

Place all the ingredients in a blender and process until smooth. Increase or decrease the amount of milk if required to obtain the correct consistency. This serving provides approximately 460 calories.

## Alternative dietary programmes

The dietary programme outlined above is a healthy eating approach that can be used alongside any type of cancer treatment. However, other dietary programmes have been designed as alternatives to orthodox cancer treatment. One example is the therapy developed by Dr Max Gerson during the early to mid twentieth century. It involves a diet that is almost vegan, apart from some fat-free yoghurt, drinking freshly prepared vegetable juices regularly throughout the day, taking a range of nutritional supplements, and embarking on a programme of detoxification. The aim is to restore biochemical integrity to the body so that healing can occur. Gerson felt this could best be achieved by regulating the sodium–potassium balance and encouraging normal thyroid function and metabolic rate.

There has been very little formal research into the Gerson Therapy or other alternative dietary cancer treatment programmes. Although it is fairly unusual for patients to choose a dietary approach *instead* of mainstream treatments, most oncologists become extremely concerned if they learn that their patients are choosing to follow such a diet and patients are more likely to opt for such diets when orthodox treatment has failed. Although many may feel that alternative cancer diets have nothing to offer and should be totally disregarded, some very positive anecdotal evidence about the Gerson Therapy exists, indicating the need for well-designed clinical trials.

## References

Argiles, J. M. 2005, Cancer-associated malnutrition, *European Journal of Oncology Nursing*, vol. **9**, no. 2, Suppl, pp. S39–50.

Balkwill, F. & Mantovani, A. 2001, Inflammation and cancer: back to Virchow? *Lancet*, vol. **357**, pp. 539–45.

Bravi, F., Bosetti, C., Scotti, L. *et al.* 2007, Food groups and renal cell carcinoma: a case-control study from Italy, *International Journal of Cancer*, vol. **120**, no. 3, pp. 681–5.

Brown, J. K. 2002, A systematic review of the evidence on symptom management of cancer-related anorexia and cachexia, *Oncology Nursing Forum*, vol. **29**, no. 3, pp. 517–30.

Chen, H. 2006, Cellular inflammatory responses: novel insights for obesity and insulin resistance, *Pharmacological Research*, vol. **53**, no. 6, pp. 469–77.

Chlebowski, R. T., Aiello, E., McTiernan. A. 2002, Weight loss in breast cancer management, *Journal of Clinical Oncology*, vol. **20**, no. 4, pp. 1128–43.

Foulstone, E., Prince, S., Zaccheo, O. *et al.* 2005, Insulin-like growth factor ligands, receptors, and binding proteins in cancer, *Journal of Pathology*, vol. **205**, no. 2, pp. 145–53.

Giovannucci, E. 2003, Nutrition, insulin, insulin-like growth factors and cancer, *Hormone and Metabolic Research*, vol. **35**, pp. 694–704.

Hardman, W. E. 2004, (n-3) fatty acids and cancer therapy, *Journal of Nutrition*, vol. **134**, no. 12 Suppl, pp. 3427S–30S.

Inoue, M., Tajima, K., Mizutani, M. *et al.* 2001, Regular consumption of green tea and the risk of breast cancer recurrence: follow-up study from the Hospital-based Epidemiologic Research Program at Aichi Cancer Center (HERPACC), Japan, *Cancer Letters*, vol. **167**, no. 2, pp. 175–82.

Ishikawa, H., Saeki, T., Otani, T. *et al.* 2006, Aged garlic extract prevents a decline of NK cell number and activity in patients with advanced cancer, *Journal of Nutrition*, vol. **136**, no. 3, Suppl. pp. 816S–20S.

Kucuk, O., Sarkar, F. H., Djuric, Z. *et al.* 2002, Effects of lycopene supplementation in patients with localized prostate cancer, *Experiental Biology and Medicine* (Maywood), vol. **227**, pp. 881–5.

McEligot, A. J., Rock, C. L., Shanks, T. G. *et al.* 1999, Comparison of serum carotenoid responses between women consuming vegetable juice and women consuming raw or cooked vegetables, *Cancer Epidemiology Biomarkers and Prevention*, vol. **8**, pp. 227–31.

Nakamura, K., Kariyazono, H., Komokata, T. *et al.* 2005, Influence of preoperative administration of omega-3 fatty acid-enriched supplement on inflammatory and immune responses in patients undergoing major surgery for cancer, *Nutrition*, vol. **21**, no. 6, pp. 639–49.

National Cancer Institute 2005, *Nutrition in Cancer Care*. PDF document available at www.cancer.gov.

Nicolson, G. L. 2005, Lipid replacement/antioxidant therapy as an adjunct supplement to reduce the adverse effects of cancer therapy and restore mitochondrial function, *Pathology and Oncology Research*, vol. **11**, no. 3, pp. 139–44.

Ohta, N., Tsujikawa, T., Nakamura, T. *et al.* 2003, A comparison of the effects of medium- and long-chain triglycerides on neutrophil stimulation in experimental ileitis, *Journal of Gastroenterology*, vol. **38**, no. 2, pp. 127–33.

Ornish, D., Weidner, G., Fair, W. *et al.* 2005, Intensive lifestyle changes may affect the progression of prostate cancer, *Journal of Urology*, vol. **174**, pp. 1065–70.

Saxe, G., Herbert, J., Carmody, J. *et al.* 2001, Can diet in conjunction with stress reduction affect the rate of increase in prostate specific antigen after biochemical recurrence of prostate cancer?, *Journal of Urology*, vol. **166**, pp. 2202–07.

Sharma, R. A., Euden, S. A., Platton, S. L. *et al.* 2004, Phase I clinical trial of oral curcumin: biomarkers of systemic activity and compliance, *Clinical Cancer Research*, vol. **10**, no. 20, pp. 6847–54.

Trichopoulou, A., Naska, A., Antoniou, A. *et al.* 2003, Vegetable and fruit: the evidence in their favour and the public health perspective. *International Journal of Vitamin and Nutrition Research*, vol. **73**, no. 2, pp. 63–9.

Chapter 21

# Reflexology

## Peter A Mackereth and Clive S O'Hara

### Summary

Reflexology is practised in many countries and has an ancient history. It involves working on the feet and besides increasing comfort, relaxation, and well-being for patients and carers, it can help to relieve cancer-related symptoms such as anxiety, pain, nausea, and lethargy. It is not unusual to find this therapy available within hospices but there have been concerns about its use when patients are receiving medical treatments such as radiotherapy and chemotherapy. This chapter reviews the theories and practice of reflexology, explores research evidence, and reports on innovative approaches to adapt treatments for patients and their carers in cancer care settings.

## Introduction

Reflexology is a popular intervention and is offered within many hospices and some specialist cancer centres (Kohn 2002). Although the mechanism of action is not fully understood, the use of reflexology techniques on patients' feet and/or hands is beginning to become accepted by nurses and medical staff as a means of reducing stress and managing anxieties related to cancer and its treatment (Hodkinson and Williams 2002). As with massage, many of its practitioners may have been told by their teachers that reflexology is contraindicated when a patient has a history of, or is being treated for, cancer; yet, there is no published evidence to support this view. Cancer is still listed as a contraindication by some awarding bodies, although this has now been corrected in the Core Curriculum for Reflexology in the UK (O'Hara 2006). It is important to acknowledge that some patients may be too poorly or fatigued to receive a treatment that in private practice can last for up to an hour. Importantly, some conventional treatments such as use of chemotherapy, radiotherapy, steroids, and analgesics may compromise peripheral sensation and skin integrity. It is therefore important for the practitioner in responding to a request for reflexology to have access to other healthcare professionals, such as a lymphoedema specialist or a podiatrist, to discuss any possible cautions or concerns. Adapting the intervention to the individual ensures that the therapy is used both effectively and safely.

## Origins, theories, and practice of reflexology

Pictorial evidence of the feet being worked for health benefits has been found in Egyptian and North American Indian art. In the early twentieth century, Dr William Fitzgerald, an American laryngologist, began investigating and writing about 'zone' therapy. In this therapy, the body is organized into 10 longitudinal zones extending along from the digits of the hands and feet, with the hypothesis that constant direct pressure on one part of the zone will potentially have an anaesthetizing effect on the entire zone (Kunz and Kunz 1993). Around the 1930s, Eunice Ingham, a nurse and physiotherapist, introduced 'alternating pressure' into the zone philosophy and produced maps of the feet. Ingham is considered to be the 'mother' of Western reflexology and she introduced training courses for health professionals and lay practitioners. One of Ingham's students, Doreen Bayly, has been credited with establishing the first British reflexology school in the late 1960s (Mackereth and O'Hara 2002).

Common to all reflexology treatments is locating 'reflex' points or areas using a map of, primarily, the feet or hands (ears and face points are sometimes used by specialists) and then treating these points with a variety of pressure techniques using the hands, thumbs, and fingers (Fig. 21.1). Relaxation techniques play a major role in the procedure, a variety of 'relaxers' introducing, interspersing, and concluding the session, which in general practice typically lasts an hour.

The reflex points are mapped to correspond to all areas of the body including specific organs. The left foot or hand relates to the left half of the body—five of the longitudinal zones—and laterally, the digits relate to the head areas, the metatarsal (carpal) region to the chest and abdomen, and the tarsal (carpal) to the pelvic area.

An original concept of reflexologists was that the alternating pressure techniques were 'breaking down deposits' on these reflexes that were impeding the 'normal flow of energy through the body'. Points were located by identifying such 'crystals' and the pressure treatment was 'breaking these down'.

More recent hypotheses involve the sensory receptors of the nervous system and locating sensitive points that indicate disordered reflexes corresponding to areas of the body affected by illness, a concept perhaps more likely to be viewed as credible by orthodox healthcare professionals.

Most reflexology practitioners work either in private clinics or in the client's home. Typically, treatments are given on a one-to-one basis, initially requiring weekly appointments. The treatment process includes cleaning the feet, when

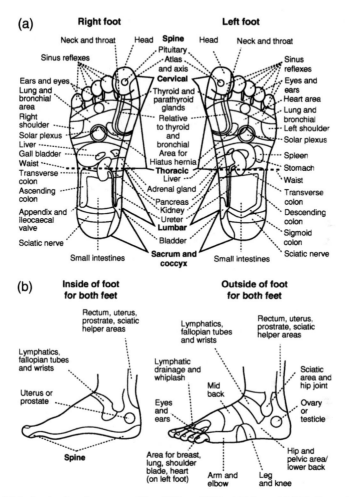

**Figure 21.1** Foot reflexology map: Clive O'Hara 1981, 1991, and 2002. Reproduced with permission of the author.

necessary, and sometimes applying minimal amounts of talc or moisturizing cream or oil to facilitate the smooth working of reflexes, some of which require precise technique. The session usually ends with a 'solar plexus (celiac ganglion) breathing' technique, which uses a specific point and the breath.

## The 'reflexology package' in the cancer care setting

Reflexology is viewed as a package rather than a set of techniques (O'Hara 2002). This concept helps to explain the suitability and popularity of reflexology in a cancer care setting. The position, and the examination of reflex points, can provide space for patients to interact with the therapist. The patient can remain fully dressed, so treatment can be both non-threatening and pleasant to receive. Reflexology can be a useful starting point from which to introduce touch as a therapy. As the therapist is usually face-to-face with the patient, there is potential for engagement in conversation, providing opportunities to share fears and anxieties related to the cancer journey (Gambles 2002; Hodkinson and Williams 2002). An overview of the 'reflexology package' is shown in Table 21.1.

## Myths

Despite an increasing amount of literature reporting the use of reflexology for patients living with cancer and its treatments, there have been concerns among some therapists and healthcare professionals that reflexology could spread cancer (Kassab and Stevensen 1996; Hodkinson 2005). There is no documented evidence to support this (MacDonald 1999; Hodkinson 2005). Whereas some schools teach that reflexology is primarily a stimulating and detoxifying treatment, current literature suggests that it is a process that balances the whole body, helping it to achieve its own equilibrium or homeostasis. A recent review of reflexology contraindications and cautions in the grey literature has highlighted a poorly founded overemphasis of the words 'stimulate' and 'increase', resulting in inappropriate conclusions about the safety of reflexology (O'Hara 2002, 2006). In addition, concern regarding working a reflex corresponding to a tumour site is also likely born from an overzealous emphasis of the word 'stimulate' rather than 'balance'.

It has also been suggested by participants in local and national reflexology study days that the claimed 'detoxification of the body' following reflexology

**Table 21.1** The 'Reflexology Package' (adapted from O'Hara in Mackereth & Tiran, 2002)

| Feature | Benefit |
| --- | --- |
| Substantial treatment duration (usually 1 hour) | Quality personal time for patient |
| One to one situation | Potential for communication |
| Face to face positioning—constant eye contact | Encourages communication |
| Tactile—continuous physical contact but practitioner is positioned at feet, at a comfortable boundary of the body | Employs therapeutic touch but—preserves personal space |
| Non-invasive technique | No equipment, pharmacological substance or need to undress |
| Can provide 'diagnostic' information about health and well-being in addition to being a therapeutic intervention | |

treatments could decrease the effectiveness of cytotoxic drugs. Again, there has been no published evidence, anecdotal or otherwise, to suggest cytotoxic drugs being rendered less effective following reflexology. Drugs are extensively researched and measured, having a specific half-life, and the above myth implies that reflexology 'stimulates' the body's elimination processes past its optimum capability (O'Hara and Marland 2004).

Another concern raised at study days is the claimed potential contamination of the therapist's hands from contact with the by-products of cytotoxic drugs through the sweat glands in the patient's skin. Cytotoxic drugs are metabolized by the liver with the by-products excreted in the faeces and urine (Dougherty and Bailey 2001). Unless the practitioner is handling body fluids or the drugs themselves, contamination through the skin is unlikely, especially if the treatment is followed by a thorough hand-washing procedure, which will be part of every competent reflexolgist's treatment plan. Again, there have been no published reports of adverse reactions from reflexology with a patient who is having chemotherapy. Indeed, patients frequently report benefits, such as the reduction in the side effects of treatment including nausea and vomiting and an increase in relaxation (Hodkinson *et al.* 2006).

Some reflexologists are wary of treating a patient who is having radiotherapy. Radiotherapists support the view that at the end of each linear accelerator treatment there is no residual radioactive material in the patient with which to contaminate others. In the case of treatments and diagnostic procedures involving implanted radioactive material, careful adherence by the reflexologist to the strict rules of contact applied to nursing staff, relatives (especially intimate partners), and carers will eliminate any need for concern (O'Hara and Marland 2004).

## Research, reflexology, and cancer care

Anecdotal evidence and some small research studies suggest that reflexology can help with many cancer-related and treatment-related symptoms, such as pain, discomfort, and lethargy. For example, Gambles *et al.* (2002) in the UK used a semi-structured questionnaire with a convenience sample ($n = 34$) of patients attending for between four and six reflexology treatments at a hospice. Patients reported helpful relief from tension and anxiety, improved well-being, feeling supported and comforted by the treatments and therapists, and being better able to cope with their diagnosis and conventional treatment.

In Australia, Grealish *et al.* (2000) used a quasi-experimental design to establish the effects of foot massage provided by nurse therapists. Hospitalized patients with cancer ($n = 87$) were randomized to receive two massages and one resting period but in three different orders or arms of the trial. Visual analogue scales were used to measure pain, nausea, and relaxation. Significant differences were found with the massage interventions, with scores demonstrating improved relaxation and reduced nausea and pain.

In America, Stephenson and Weinrich (2000) completed a crossover trial in which patients ($n = 23$) with lung or breast cancer were randomized to receive (a) 30 minutes of reflexology followed by a 30-minute control time after a 2-day break or (b) 30 minutes of control time, 2-day break, and then 30 minutes of reflexology. There was a significant decrease in anxiety reported following the reflexology treatment but effects on pain reduction were less apparent.

More recently, in the UK, Smith (2002) investigated the benefits of reflexology for women with breast cancer ($n = 150$) receiving radiotherapy and reported significant differences for both reflexology and foot massage (given by the same therapist) compared with standard care in some subscales of a mood scale and fatigue checklist. For reflexology, there was a trend for a possible effect on lymphocyte activity worthy of further investigation.

A skilled and experienced practitioner can adapt treatments to work safely and potently to suit the individual in a wide range of situations. There are recognized cautions and conditions of which the therapist will need to be aware in order to adapt the treatment, for example, deep-vein thrombosis, neuropathy, low platelet count, and lymphoedema (Tavares 2003). Absolute contraindications are usually those surrounding consent, for example, where a patient is not capable or competent to give consent. Infection risk may also need to be considered if the patient has a severely compromised immune system (O'Hara 2006). If in doubt, the reflexologist must always consult with the patient's medical and nursing team.

There are many factors affecting the nature of the reflexes of the feet and their condition must be taken into consideration when assessing a patient and planning a treatment. Drugs such as strong analgesics, hypnotics, steroids, tranquillizers, and cytotoxics can alter sensation in the feet causing reduced sensitivity or occasionally hypersensitivity. Chronic illness and emotional and physical pain can also affect sensitivity in reflexes, as can tumours of the central nervous system, neuropathy, and other non-cancer–related conditions such as multiple sclerosis and stroke (Tavares 2003).

## Adaptations

Reflexology can be given virtually anywhere within reason, provided the feet, and sometimes hands, are accessible. Patients can be treated in a clinical setting or at home, whether in bed, an armchair, or wheelchair, in the garden on a warm day, or in a specially designated relaxation room. Some patients may prefer their families or partner to be present. Indeed, seeing their loved one having therapy can be relaxing in itself for carers. Reflexology does not always necessitate being treated behind hospital curtains or in a treatment room, but a quiet and pleasant environment can facilitate deeper relaxation. A patient with severe weight changes, poor nutrition, and poor skin integrity may be at risk of developing pressure sores, so care must be taken with both positioning and length of treatment.

A breathless patient may be more comfortable when sitting upright or in a high side-lying position (requires an adjustable backrest and support pillows). If available, a bed table can be used with pillows, with the patient leaning forward in the orthopnoeic position. Care must be taken not to overly engage a breathless patient in conversation. In many situations, the patient is most likely to be treated in a chair by the bedside or in bed. It is important that practitioners ensure that the patient is comfortable while not compromising on their own posture.

## Innovative techniques

Some reflexologists use deep-pressure techniques and sometimes even hard implements to treat reflex points. Aside from risk to underlying soft tissue and fragile skin, these could also cause unnecessary distress and pain. Light gentle touch is commonly used with patients in palliative and cancer care settings. Not only is it is much safer in terms of reducing trauma to skin and soft tissue but it can be useful in managing physical symptoms. Descriptors of some innovative reflexology techniques, summarized from the work of colleagues and the authors of this chapter (Hodkinson *et al.* 2006), are shown in Table 21.2.

### Case study

Malcolm, aged 64 years, had been treated for carcinoma of the rectum with surgery and chemotherapy prior to attending the hospice with recurrence of carcinoma, and liver and lung metastases. In this setting, he began having reflexology, reporting improvements in his symptoms such as a reduction in pain and fatigue, and for help in managing the side effects of medication, as well as providing time to discuss his situation.

In the final 6 months of Malcolm's life, his wife also started to receive reflexology. Doreen reported that it had helped her adjust to leaving work to care for Malcolm, this being triggered by a fall when he was at home on his own. Their respect for, and eagerness to receive, reflexology was demonstrated, on what was to be their final session together, by Doreen pushing Malcolm's wheelchair over a mile uphill to the cancer support centre, despite the rain and his failing heath. Malcolm was admitted to the hospice again a week later. The day before he died, Doreen and the hospice reflexologist worked alongside each other treating a foot each, a significant event that provided benefits for all involved. Doreen continues to receive reflexology and helps in fundraising events for both the hospice and cancer support centre.

This case study also shows how reflexology can be an appropriate intervention when all other treatment has stopped. The resulting closure is invaluable for the therapist as well as the patient and carer, especially when they may have been the primary practitioner and played a major role in the patient's journey.

**Table 21.2** Innovative techniques in reflexology

| Techniques | Description |
|---|---|
| Precision Reflexology<br>Developed by Pru Miskin and Jan Williams | Gentle linking of specific reflexology points. Techniques can involve stillness and focus. Specific areas of the body such as the endocrine system and chakras of body are treated. Links can also involve bony structures and organs of the body |
| AirReflexology©<br>Developed by Edwina Hodkinson and Barbara Cook | Involves combining reflexology theory and map to provide 'off the skin' or energy field reflexology |
| HypnoReflexology©<br>Developed by Peter Mackereth and Paula Maycock | Deep relaxation techniques using breath work, pressure point work combined with hypnotherapy techniques, i.e., controlled use of the voice, safe space, and anchoring techniques to help with anxiety, needle phobia, pain, and nausea |
| Creative Relaxation Reflexology<br>Developed by Barbara Cook | Combines gentle reflexology with creative imagery and visualization |
| 4-Hands Holding Reflexology<br>(Mackereth et al, 2000) | Involves two qualified therapists working together with a patient. Treatments are usually shorter and can involve working the feet and hands together |

## Working with carers

A diagnosis of cancer can be very distressing, not only for the patient but for the family, friends, and colleagues. It may reduce their energy levels and increase anxiety. Receiving a reflexology treatment can help carers to take time out and to focus on their own needs. It can also create opportunities for carers to talk about their feelings, to help them to manage their own anxiety and stress, and to deal with issues that they feel unable to talk about with their loved ones (Hodkinson and Williams 2002). Carers may have health concerns of their own, precipitated or exacerbated by the burden of caring. Reflexology can help in coping and managing such problems and provide a safe environment in which to receive support.

## Summary of recommendations

In conclusion, this chapter has explored approaches to reflexology that are both innovative and mindful of patients' symptoms and safety. In order to skilfully adapt the treatment for cancer care settings, it is important to recognize that reflexologists require additional training, support, and supervision (O'Hara 2006).

- Working closely with healthcare professionals is important to ensure treatments take account of medical concerns. For example, if lymphoedema is present, it is essential to seek advice, and where possible assessment, from a specialist prior to treatment

- Reflexology treatments can be adapted to ensure safety, comfort, and effectiveness. Consider offering short and gentle sessions for patients with fatigue or those undergoing chemotherapy

- It is important to always consider how clients can be involve in the treatment and empowered. Patients (and carers) can be taught simple techniques with skilled supervision

- Hands or ears can be considered if the feet are inaccessible and affected by cancer and its treatment

- It is important to evaluate and develop best practice. Further research within cancer care settings would be helpful to evaluate the longer-term effects and to assess innovative approaches to reflexology.

## References

Dougherty, L. & Bailey, C. 2001, Chemotherapy. In *Cancer Care in Context*, (eds) J. Corner, C. Bailey, Blackwell Science, Oxford.

Gambles, M., Crooke, M. & Wilkinson, S. 2002, Evaluation of a hospice based reflexology service: a qualitative audit of patient perceptions, *European Journal of Oncology Nursing*, vol. **6**, no. 1, pp. 37–44.

Grealish, L., Lomasney, A. & Whiteman, B. 2000, Foot massage: a nursing intervention to modify the distressing symptoms of pain and nausea in patients hospitalised with cancer, *Cancer Nursing*, vol. **23**, no. 3, pp. 237–43.

Griffiths, P. 1996, Reflexology. In *The Nurse's Handbook of Complementary Therapies*, (ed) D. Rankin-Box, Churchill Livingstone, London.

Hodkinson, E. & Williams, J. 2002, Enhancing quality of life for people in palliative care settings. In *Clinical Reflexology: a guide for health professionals*, (eds) P. Mackereth, D. Tiran, Elsevier Science, London.

Hodkinson, E. 2005, Reflexology for people with cancer. *Reflexions*, June issue, 2–5.

Hodkinson, E., Mackereth, P. & Cook, B. 2006, Creative approaches to reflexology. In *Massage & Bodywork: adapting therapies for cancer care*, (eds) P. Mackereth, C. Carter, Elsevier Science, London.

Kassab, S. & Stevensen, C. 1996, Common misunderstandings about complementary therapies for people with cancer, *Complementary Therapies in Nursing and Midwifery*, vol. **2**, 3, pp. 62–65.

Kohn, M. 2002, *Directory of Complementary Therapy Services in the UK*. Macmillan Cancer Relief, London.

Kunz, K. & Kunz, B. 1993, *The Complete Guide to Foot Reflexology (Revised)*. Kunz & Kunz, Albuquerque, New Mexico.

MacDonald, G. 1999, *Medicine Hands: Massage Therapy for People with Cancer*. Findhorne Press, Tallahassee FL.

Mackereth, P. & O'Hara, C. 2002, Appreciating preparatory and continuing education. In *Clinical Reflexology: A Guide for Health Professionals*, (eds) P. Mackereth, D. Tiran, Elsevier Science, London.

O'Hara, C. 2002, Challenging the 'rules' of reflexology. In *Clinical reflexology: A Guide for Health Professionals*, (eds) P. Mackereth, D. Tiran, Elsevier Science, London.

O'Hara, C. & Marland, L. 2004, Am I at risk when treating people with cancer? In CRN 13, Manchester, England.

O'Hara, C. S. 2006, *Core Curriculum for Reflexology*. Douglas Barry Publications, London.

Smith, G. 2002, A randomised controlled clinical trial of reflexology in breast cancer patients, to reduce fatigue resulting from radiotherapy to the breast and chest wall. Unpublished PhD thesis, University of Liverpool.

Stephenson, N. L. N. & Weinrich, S. P. 2000, The effects of foot reflexology on anxiety and pain in patients with breast and lung cancer, *Oncology Nursing Forum*, vol. 27, no. 1, pp. 67–72.

Tavares, M. 2003, *National Guidelines for the Use of Complementary Therapies in Supportive and Palliative Care*. The Foundation for Integrated Health, London.

Chapter 22

# Relaxation, visualization, and hypnotherapy

Leslie G Walker, Donald M Sharp, Andrew A Walker, and Mary B Walker

## Summary

A systematic review of the use of complementary and alternative medicine in patients with cancer reported an average use of 31% across 13 countries, although the range was wide (7–64%) (Ernst and Cassileth 1998). Many patients experience distress following the diagnosis of cancer and wish to pursue methods that they believe might help them to feel more relaxed and in control, as well as minimize treatment side effects. This chapter focuses on three such interventions: relaxation therapy, visualization, and hypnotherapy. They all share some non-specific factors including a healing ritual, a helping relationship, hope, suggestion, and expectation of change. However, there are a number of important theoretical and practical differences that are described below.

## Relaxation therapy

The 'relaxation response' is an integrated psychobiological phenomenon that is characterized by feelings of physical and mental relaxation. In particular, it is associated with reduced heart rate, peripheral vasodilatation, diaphragmatic breathing, increased alpha activity in the brain, and reduced muscle tone. It can usefully be considered to be the opposite of the 'fight–flight' response, which is one of the body's automatic and usually adaptive responses to an acute severe threat.

There are many ways of inducing the relaxation response but two landmarks were the development of progressive muscular relaxation training methods by Jacobson (1929) and cue-controlled relaxation by Suinn and Richardson in the 1960s.

Progressive muscular relaxation training involves a systematic series of exercises designed to relax all the main muscles in the body. Typically, the exercises begin with the fingers and hands and then move to the arms, shoulders, neck, scalp, face, eyes, tongue, chest, abdomen, back, hips, legs, feet, and toes. To take the hands as an example, the person would be asked to make a fist for several seconds, notice the tension, and then relax the muscles. This is usually repeated once or twice in an attempt to produce 'rebound relaxation'.

Cue-controlled relaxation involves similar procedures to progressive muscular relaxation training in the initial stages (Suinn and Richardson 1971). In addition, at the point when tension is released, the subject is asked to say out loud, or to think, a phrase such as 'one-two-three-relax!'. With repetition, and by association, these trigger words become a cue (or conditioned stimulus) for switching on the relaxation response.

Some approaches to inducing the relaxation response include special breathing exercises. Patients are taught to inhale slowly and deeply (diaphragmatic breathing) rather than quickly and shallowly (thoracic breathing).

Mental exercises are usually incorporated into relaxation training. These often involve the use of 'special place imagery', whereby the subject is asked to recall a time and place when he or she felt particularly calm, in control, and relaxed. The subject is invited to become so absorbed in this memory that it seems as real as possible.

With cue-controlled relaxation, the intention is that the subject will learn to switch on the relaxation response when and where he or she wishes. This could be, for example, before, during, or after radiotherapy or chemotherapy.

## Indications

There is evidence that relaxation therapy can help many patients cope better with various aspects of cancer and its treatment, as witnessed by reduced anxiety, more positive mood, and improved quality of life. A number of randomized controlled trials have found that relaxation therapy can ameliorate chemotherapy side effects, particularly anticipatory nausea and vomiting, help treatment-related anxiety, and reduce acute pain (Luebbert *et al.* 2001). It can also be used as part of an intervention to help with procedural distress caused by needles or enclosed spaces such as magnetic resonance scanners (Anderson and Walker 2002).

## Contraindications and cautions

It is important to advise patients that they should avoid tensing specific muscles if this causes pain, for example because of recent surgery or joint disease. In our opinion, except in the hands of the most experienced mental health practitioners, relaxation therapy should not be used in patients who have a history of psychosis or are currently psychotic. In these individuals, any procedure that blurs the boundaries between fantasy and reality could be harmful.

Relaxation methods should be used with caution in patients with clinically significant depression. Relaxation therapy is not the treatment of choice for depression and a consequence of offering relaxation training to a depressed patient might be that he or she failed to seek a more appropriate treatment. Moreover, depressed patients often have impaired concentration and low self-esteem; they may therefore find it difficult to learn relaxation techniques and their slow progress may simply add to their feelings of inadequacy.

Relaxation-induced anxiety, or even panic, occurs very rarely during the initial stages of learning to relax, probably related to a self-perceived loss of control. Depending on circumstances, the patient may or may not be advised to persevere.

## Practical considerations

Progressive muscular relaxation and cue-controlled relaxation can be taught through live sessions with a therapist, by listening to audio recordings, or a combination of both. Most individuals find that audio recordings, which they can use in the comfort and privacy of their own home at a time convenient to them, are more than adequate. If patients are having difficulty learning relaxation, however, a few live sessions can be beneficial in pinpointing the nature of the difficulties and helping the patient to overcome these.

As far as the frequency of practice is concerned, there is little sound research on which to base advice. Our experience is that encouraging patients to practise at least once per day during the first few weeks produces better results than a lower frequency. In a study of 96 women with locally advanced breast cancer, half of whom were randomized to relaxation and guided imagery during their neo-adjuvant chemotherapy (Walker *et al.* 1999), we found that approximately 50% of patients practise relaxation less than once a day on average, and 20% of these even less frequently. Evidently, a significant number of patients either will not, or cannot, practise regularly and it is important that they are not made to feel guilty because of this.

We use relaxation, and the other two methods described subsequently, in the context of a comprehensive Oncology Health Service, where all patients receive a high level of information and support. All patients are screened for clinically significant distress. All our staff have been trained to diagnose psychiatric morbidity and a range of evidence-based interventions, psychotherapeutic and pharmacological, are available if indicated (Walker *et al.* 2003).

## Evaluation and conclusions

There is evidence that relaxation methods can be beneficial in coping with various aspects of the diagnosis and treatment of cancer. However, they are certainly not a panacea and there are a group of patients who for one reason or another are unwilling to practise these methods.

## Visualization

The importance of visual images to *Homo sapiens* is well illustrated by the discovery of paintings in the Lion's Cave in South Africa, estimated to be 43,000 years old.

The Greek philosopher Aristotle is reported to have said, 'The soul never thinks without a picture'. More recently, the greatest physicist of the last century, Albert Einstein, said in an interview that 'Imagination is more important than education'. The billions of pounds spent annually by the advertising industry on visual images testify to the perceived power of images in altering feelings, attitudes, and behaviours.

The term 'visualization' can be used in two ways. First, it can be used to describe a variety of procedures whereby therapists assist patients to feel more relaxed using visual images. For example, patients may be invited to visualize, as vividly as they can, a time and a place when they felt relaxed, calm, confident, and 'in control', and to re-experience these feelings as intensely as they can. In addition to recalling the visual aspects of the memory, they may also be encouraged to recall auditory, tactile, kinaesthetic, and tactile stimuli that they associate with this relaxing 'special place'. Used in this way, visualization is a very common component of both relaxation therapy and hypnotherapy.

Second, visualization can refer to a more specific procedure whereby patients visualize their bodies' own natural defences, for example, their white blood cells destroying cancer cells or in some other way promoting health (Simonton *et al.* 1980). It is in this sense that we use the term here. Some patients use a 'fighting spirit' metaphor and visualize, for example, a soldier with a bayonet attaching a cluster of cancer cells. Others prefer to visualize a phagocytic process, for example, fish-like creatures swimming in blood and lymph looking for a primary tumour or occult metastases.

Visualization is often combined with relaxation because relaxation is thought to facilitate more vivid imagery. In our study of women being treated for locally advanced breast cancer (Walker *et al.* 1999), 96 subjects were randomized to a high level of support in our unit or to a similar high level of support plus relaxation and visualization. Progressive muscular relaxation and cue-controlled relaxation were taught using live training sessions as well as audio recordings. Patients were given a portfolio of 10 coloured drawings to help them generate ideas as to how they might visualize their white blood cells working to improve their future health (examples of the images used are shown in Colour plates 6 and 7). Compared to the comparison group, those randomized to relaxation therapy and visualization reported more positive mood, better quality of life, and improved coping. Moreover, analysis of blood samples taken on 11 occasions over a 37-week period (during which time the women underwent neo-adjuvant chemotherapy, surgery and radiotherapy, as well as hormone therapy) showed more mature T cells, more activated T cells, and a higher number of a subset of natural killer cells that are thought to have anti-tumour activity. Interestingly, in the women randomized to relaxation and imagery, self-ratings of imagery vividness correlated highly with killer cell activity following chemotherapy and 37 weeks after the diagnosis.

## Indications

The effect of this type of visualization on its own has not been well studied. Currently, we are evaluating the effects of relaxation and guided imagery, alone and in combination, in 150 patients with colorectal cancer.

In combination with relaxation, visualization does seem to improve quality of life, mood, and coping abilities, perhaps by increasing feelings of self-control, or 'self-efficacy'.

## Contraindications and cautions

As for relaxation on its own, psychosis should probably be considered a contraindication and imagery should be used with caution in patients who are significantly depressed. In addition, there are three specific considerations for visualization.

First, if patients believe that their cancer has been cured, it is obviously inappropriate for them to visualize their white blood cells destroying cancer cells. However, some patients still feel vulnerable about the possibility of recurrence, in which case a surveillance metaphor might be appropriate. For example, they may wish to visualize a metaphorical police force on patrol, able to deal with cancerous cells if the need should arise. It is important, however, that this does not become a preoccupation.

Second, some patients cope well using a 'minimization strategy' that involves a conscious attempt to keep cancer and its implications at the back of one's mind. Although not everybody can use this strategy, for those who can, it has been shown to be associated with a good quality of life. Asking such patients to practise visualization might serve as an unhelpful reminder of their illness.

Finally, the 'fighting spirit' cannot be sustained indefinitely and it is very important to make sure that patients do not have unrealistic expectations about having to 'feel positive', as this could lead to a sense of failure and inadequacy.

## Practical considerations

Neither the optimal frequency of practice nor the effectiveness of live versus recorded instructions is known.

In our experience, it is helpful for patients to develop their own images, rather than adopt standardized ones. Moreover, they may wish to use different images at different points in their treatment. In practice, we find that good images meet two criteria: first, the patient feels comfortable with the image (in other words, the image is 'ego-syntonic'); second, it is 'psycho-logical' (in other words, it seems logical to the patient, even if it is not scientifically logical).

## Evaluation and conclusions

Under certain circumstances, visualization would seem to be a helpful treatment. However, most of the research has studied its effects in conjunction with relaxation therapy. Further research is needed to clarify acceptability and effectiveness on its own.

# Hypnotherapy

According to a recent consensus statement (British Psychological Society 2001):

> The term 'Hypnosis' denotes an interaction between one person, 'the Hypnotist', and another person or people, 'the Subject' or 'Subjects'. In this interaction, the hypnotist attempts to influence the subjects' perceptions, feelings, thinking and behaviour by asking them to concentrate on ideas and images that may evoke the intended effects. The verbal communications that the hypnotist uses to achieve these effects are termed as 'suggestions' ... Subjects may learn to go through the hypnotic procedures on their own, and this is termed 'self-hypnosis' (p. 3).

Hypnosis is usually associated with narrowing of attention, increased suggestibility, inner-absorption, and detachment from immediate realities. Contrary to popular belief, unless amnesia is suggested during the session, most patients are able to recall their hypnotic experiences in considerable detail.

Clinical hypnotherapy usually involves the following stages:

♦ Preparation of the patient in terms of addressing any concerns and giving information

♦ Induction

♦ Deepening

♦ Therapeutic work (e.g. ego-strengthening, de-conditioning, rehearsal in imagination, anchoring)

♦ Termination

♦ Debriefing.

Relaxation is usually used for the induction procedure. Typically, patients are then invited to experience various phenomena, for example, arm heaviness, and this is coupled with suggestions of 'trance' deepening. Once the therapist is satisfied that an appropriate mental state has been achieved, therapeutic procedures are carried out.

In the 1980s, we developed a novel intervention for chemotherapy-related nausea and vomiting. The intervention included hypnotherapy, relaxation training, and 'nausea management training' (Walker *et al.* 1988; Walker 2004). Nausea management training involves teaching progressive muscular relaxation and cue-controlled relaxation. Following hypnotic induction, patients are asked to experience treatment-related side effects by remembering their last treatment or some other trigger. They are then given practice in 'relaxing away' the feelings of anxiety and nausea. Ego-strengthening suggestions to enhance self-efficacy are also given; patients are told that as they became more skilled in applying their relaxation, they will be able to feel more relaxed, more confident, and more in control whenever they wish.

In one of our studies, we randomized 63 patients with Hodgkin's disease or non-Hodgkin's lymphoma to medical treatment for chemotherapy side effects, medical treatment plus relaxation therapy, or medical treatment plus nausea management training (Walker 2004). Both psychological interventions had beneficial effects on treatment side effects. Surprisingly, when the patients were followed up, those who had been randomized either to relaxation or nausea management training had survived significantly longer, even when other prognostic factors were taken into account in a multivariate analysis. This survival benefit was restricted to those who scored high on a measure of social conformity, itself an independent negative prognostic factor for survival. The study was not designed to detect differences in survival and clearly further research is required to determine whether the findings can be replicated.

## Indications

Combined with cognitive-behavioural principles, hypnotherapy can be effective in the rapid treatment of needle phobia and claustrophobia (which may cause problems when, for example, scans or radiotherapy involve fixation to a table or application of a mask). There is also good evidence that it can be beneficial for anxiety, nausea, and vomiting associated with chemotherapy, particularly anticipatory nausea and vomiting. It can aid cue-controlled relaxation and, if ego-strengthening suggestions are given, it can enhance feelings of self-efficacy. There is also evidence that it can be helpful for pain control, particularly where the pain is acute.

## Contraindications and cautions

As with relaxation, unless the practitioner is highly experienced, hypnotherapy should not be used in patients with a history of psychosis and caution is required for those with clinically significant depression. It has been claimed that hypnotherapy can increase the risk of suicide in severely depressed patients, although this is difficult to prove.

Because of the intense nature of the therapist–patient relationship, caution is also required for patients with certain types of personality disorder, particularly if the therapist and patient are of different genders.

Occasionally, patients will abreact during hypnotherapy and it is important that the therapist knows how to deal with this if it happens.

## Practical considerations

Although the line between relaxation and guided imagery on the one hand and hypnotherapy on the other is hard to draw in practice, debate about the professional qualifications and appropriate training for practitioners has centred around hypnotherapy. Wide-ranging views have been expressed.

The view of the British Psychological Society is:

> Training in hypnosis should only be undertaken on the understanding that hypnosis is a set of procedures that may be used to augment one of the established psychological therapies or to facilitate psychological procedures in medicine and dentistry. Training in hypnosis for the purpose of applying it therapeutically should, therefore, only be undertaken by individuals who already possess, or are in the process or acquiring, professional qualifications and experience in understanding and treating those problems for which they intend using hypnosis (British Psychological Society 2001).

In our unit, we have institutionally agreed protocols for the use of hypnotherapy. These indicate the psychological screening and assessment procedures to be used by nurses and psychologists. Based on the contraindications and cautions described above, the protocol details the circumstances in which it is appropriate for hypnotherapy to be carried out and the circumstances in which the opinion of a more experienced colleague should be sought.

## Evaluation and conclusions

Hypnotherapy has a useful part to play in the management of various cancer-related problems, particularly when a rapid resolution is required. It is important that therapists undergo appropriate training and supervision before using hypnotherapeutic methods for clinical purposes.

## Case history

Ms A, a middle-aged woman, was referred because of severe chemotherapy-related nausea. She had recently undergone a wide local excision with axillary sampling for breast cancer and had received three of a planned eight cycles of adjuvant combination chemotherapy. Despite optimal anti-emetic medication, post-chemotherapy nausea had become increasingly distressing and on the last occasion had persisted for more than a week after chemotherapy, causing her to spend much of the time in bed. She had developed anticipatory (conditioned) nausea: simply talking about chemotherapy was enough to make her feel sick. She had not vomited either before or after chemotherapy.

As a child, Ms A had suffered from travel sickness and in adulthood even moderate amounts of alcohol would make her vomit (both known risk factors for anticipatory nausea).

Significantly, Ms A perceived chemotherapy in negative terms: it was a 'toxic' foreign substance that caused alopecia and vomiting and was associated with 'cancer', which in turn was associated with death (several relatives had died from cancer following chemotherapeutic treatment). Moreover, the chemotherapy made her feel 'out of control'.

A full mental state examination revealed no significant abnormalities.

## Session one (mental state examination, psychosocial history, and first treatment)

1. *Reframing.* Using cognitive behavioural techniques, we helped her to view chemotherapy in positive terms. Chemotherapy became her 'friend' because it was part of the 'team' that would ensure that she had the best-possible health in the future.

2. *Relaxation therapy.* Ms A was given an explanation and rationale for the use of progressive muscular and cue-controlled relaxation. An audio recording was issued for twice-daily practice, provided she did not feel nauseous. (There is some evidence that listening to a recording can become a conditioned stimulus for nausea if the patient listens to it while feeling nauseous in the early training stages.)

3. *Nausea management training.* Ms A was given information about nausea management training and there was discussion about the possible benefits of hypnotherapy.

## Session two (7 days later)

The patient had practised the relaxation exercises as agreed at the first session and had decided that she would like to receive hypnotherapy.

1. *Hypnotherapy* was induced using live relaxation; deepening was achieved by the use of special place imagery and direct suggestions.

2. *Nausea management training.* Ms A was asked to bring on a feeling of nausea in whatever way she chose and to signal with her hand when this had reached a mildly distressing level. She was able to do this almost instantly with an intensity of 6 on a 10-point scale of nausea. She was then asked to rub her abdomen gently and, as she did so, to visualize and feel the relaxation flowing inwards, soothing, calming, and refreshing her. She was asked to stop rubbing when the nausea had completely disappeared, which it did in approximately 20 seconds. The procedure was repeated twice with good effect.

3. *Ego strengthening.* While she was still hypnotized, we pointed out how by using the power of her mind she had been able both to induce nausea and to eliminate it. She was becoming more in control of how she felt moment by moment. Moreover, as she continued to practise relaxation, she would become more skilled at relaxing when and where she wished, especially around the time of chemotherapy. Consequently, she would be more in control of her feelings, moment by moment.

4. *Hypnotherapy* was then terminated.

Ms A was then taught autohypnosis using eye-roll induction and 'anchoring' techniques and she was asked to practise this daily instead of listening to the relaxation recordings.

At the end of the session, we discussed 'olfactory re-conditioning', a technique we have been developing over a number of years. Smells often become conditioned stimuli for nausea. Re-conditioning involves helping patients to identify 'counter-nausea' smells, which have a refreshing effect. Ms A found that lavender had such an effect and she was asked to smell lavender oil as often as she could each day before her next cycle of chemotherapy. If she felt nauseous before, during, or after her next cycle of chemotherapy, she was to smell the lavender oil and to practise autohypnosis.

## Session three (a week after her fourth cycle of chemotherapy)

Ms A began by saying that she was absolutely delighted with her progress. She had experienced virtually no nausea following her last cycle of chemotherapy and did not have to stay in bed. She felt more in control and very pleased about what she had achieved.

A further session of hypnotherapy was carried out along similar lines to the first session, except that in addition to nausea management training, hypnotically induced nausea was eliminated by asking her to smell the lavender oil.

With the help of one further session of hypnotherapy, support, and the continuing use of autohypnosis, Ms A was able to complete all eight cycles of chemotherapy.

## Conclusions

Relaxation, visualization, and hypnotherapy are related interventions that can play a useful part in helping patients cope with various aspects of the diagnosis and treatment of cancer and a reasonable evidence base exists to support their use. Like drugs, these interventions have indications, contraindications, and cautions. It is important that practitioners are familiar with these before attempting to utilize them in clinical practice.

A number of important practical questions regarding their application in clinical practice remain unanswered and research directed towards answering these questions merits relatively high priority by cancer research funding bodies (Redd *et al.* 2001). None of the interventions described in this chapter is a panacea; however, all have an evidence-based part to play in the practice of oncology in the twenty-first century.

## References

Anderson J and Walker LG (2002). Psychological aspects of MRI breast screening in women at high risk of breast cancer. In R Warren and A Coultard, eds.. *Breast MRI in Practice*. Martin Dunitz, London.

Ernst E and Cassileth BR (1998). The prevalence of complementary/alternative medicine in cancer: a systematic review. *Cancer*, **83**, 777–782.

British Psychological Society (2001). *The Nature of Hypnosis: A report prepared by a Working Party at the request of the Professional Affairs Board of The British Psychological Society*. British Psychological Society, Leicester.

Jacobson, E (1929). *Progressive Relaxation*. The University of Chicago Monographs in Medicine, pp. xiii, 429. University of Chicago Press, Chicago.

Luebbert K, Dahme B, Hasenbring M (2001). The effectiveness of relaxation training in reducing treatment-related symptoms and improving emotional adjustment in acute non-surgical cancer treatment: a meta-analytical review. *Psycho Oncology*, **10**, 490–502.

Redd WH, Montgomery GH and DuHamel KM (2001). Behavioral intervention for cancer treatment side effects. *Journal of the National Cancer Institute*, **93**, 810–823.

Simonton OC, Matthews-Simonton S and Sparks TF (1980). Psychological intervention in the treatment of cancer. *Psychosomatics*, **21**, 226–233.

Suinn RM and Richardson F (1971). Anxiety management training: a non-specific behaviour therapy program for anxiety control. *Behavior Therapy*, **2**, 498–410.

Walker LG, Dawson AA, Pollet SM, Ratcliffe MA, Hamilton L (1988). Hypnotherapy for chemotherapy side effects. *British Journal of Experimental and Clinical Hypnosis*, **5**, 79–82.

Walker LG, Walker MB, Heys SD *et al.* (1999). The psychological, clinical and pathological effects of relaxation training and imagery during primary chemotherapy. *British Journal of Cancer*, **80**, 262–268.

Walker LG (2004). Hypnotherapeutic insights and interventions: a cancer odyssey. *Contemporary Hypnosis*, **21**, 35–45.

Walker LG, Walker MB, Sharp DM (2003). The organisation of psychosocial support within palliative care. In M Lloyd-Williams, ed. *Psychosocial Issues in Palliative Care*. Oxford University Press, Oxford.

Chapter 23

# The spiritual dimension

Alastair J Cunningham and
Claire VI Edmonds

## Summary

The suffering cancer induces is ultimately psychological and stems from fears about likely outcome of the disease. Healing, the relief from suffering, is about changing such fears towards peace and acceptance. Patients are often left to wrestle with their fears alone but many can be helped to gain a degree of mastery over their mental state. One method of intervention involves psychospiritual therapy and a comprehensive stepwise program of this kind, the Healing Journey, is described here. This draws on modern Western psychology but to an even greater extent on the spiritual or wisdom traditions of mankind. The 'journey' of healing becomes a search for meaning. Quotes from 'graduates' illustrate that it is entirely feasible to help people with life-threatening disease to reach a profound degree of active acceptance of their situation.

## Introduction

Cancer is an existential problem, generally treated by Western healthcare as a purely physical one. Much of the suffering associated with cancer comes from anticipation of premature death (Ryan *et al.* 2005; Bultz and Carlson 2006; Vachon 2006). Perhaps because of a sense that little can be done to alleviate this fear, patients tend to be left to handle it alone, unless they seek out a counsellor or support group or fall into a clinically recognizable depression. Yet our mortality, premature or not, has been the concern of the great spiritual traditions for millennia and much of what they have taught us can be applied to assisting people with cancer.

This chapter is about helping patients with cancer through group psychological and spiritual therapy. It does not claim to be a comprehensive review of the literature but is a point of view based on some 25 years of conducting a large clinical program for outpatients and researching the value of this to them and their family members. Table 23.1 summarizes the understanding we have arrived at and compares this with the views that appear to inform current practice of oncology in most settings.

**Table 23.1** Lessons learned from a 25-year psychospiritual program for patients with cancer

| Current (medical research) literature | Our experience with a 25-year program |
|---|---|
| Existential concerns are of relatively minor importance in cancer, compared with symptom management | Existential questions ('Am I going to die prematurely?') are of major concern to many patients with cancer and may cause most of their suffering |
| Where existential concerns are addressed, this may be done by offering:<br>◆ support and comfort<br>◆ religious ideas<br>◆ meaning making ideas (e.g., using the concepts of existential philosophy) | While all of these approaches may be useful, it is possible to go beyond the purely psychological and social construction of meaning. With help, many patients learn that they are accepted unreservedly into a transcendent, non-material, loving divine order. This is spiritual experience |
| Spiritual issues need be addressed only at the end of life (in the last few weeks) | Spiritual issues are of vital importance from the time a life-threatening disease is is diagnosed (and before—but few are motivated to pursue them then!) |
| **Spiritual therapy** | |
| (a) Spiritual assistance can be provided only by religious professionals or spiritual assistance can be provided by any interested healthcare professional | (a) It needs to be provided, in a non-sectarian way, by persons with psychological and spiritual training and their own authentic experience |
| (b) Spiritual interventions can be derived from:<br>◆ conventional psychology<br>◆ religious practices<br>◆ 'western' secular philosophies<br>◆ the current scientific literature on spirituality and healing | (b) The experts on spirituality are the mystics, East and West. Their views and experiences (available through many books, workshops, and spiritual centres) are therefore the most relevant for developing interventions. The scientific literature lags far behind in its understanding of spirituality and healing |
| (c) It is sufficient to discuss ideas associated with spirituality | (c) It is necessary, if they are to be helpful, that spiritual ideas be internalized, and that spiritual practices be integrated into life |
| (d) Spiritual issues can be adequately addressed as a small part of a single brief program (e.g., 8-weekly sessions) of psychological therapy | (d) Spiritual ideas need time and effort at least equivalent to purely psychological issues. They may be offered as components of an expanded group program (see text) |

**Table 23.1** (*cont.*)

| | |
|---|---|
| (e) Spiritual ideas and practices can be introduced from the first session of therapy | (e) This is effective for some but many people need time to learn some mind-quieting techniques, such as relaxation and meditation, before they can begin to acquire spiritual experience |

**Research**

| | |
|---|---|
| Spirituality is simply one dimension of psychological experience. It may be treated like any other psychological variable | Spirituality addresses a domain beyond the material; i.e., its study leads to a different view of reality. Conventional study methods (self-report of experience) may be used, but standard concepts like 'causality' may not apply |
| Testing the value of 'spiritual therapy' must be done within the guidelines of medical research, i.e., treat it like a drug: | For many reasons, the importance of spirituality cannot be adequately addressed in this way: |
| (a) RCTs[1] of therapy versus no therapy are the ultimate test | (a) people vary enormously in their interest and experience: thus RCTs may be misleading (group means do not capture individual potential). Exploratory research and qualitative analysis of individual patterns are more appropriate at this stage |
| (b) Outcomes concern quality of life, assessed by standard self-report instruments | (b) Asking patients to score aspects of their quality of life through paper and pencil questionnaires captures very little of their experience. Observational and interview-type data are needed |
| (c) Prolongation of life is not a possible outcome of spiritual help | (c) The possibility that life may be prolonged by spiritual therapy must be kept open |
| (d) 'Contextual' variables, such as the therapists' personality and experience, the therapy setting and the expectations created, are unimportant | (d) Contextual variables may be decisive; hence the need for exploratory research until they are better understood |

[1] RCTs, Randomized controlled trials

# Helping patients to cope with the fear of death

There seem to be three main approaches: support, existential counselling, and psychospiritual therapy. Support groups for patients with cancer are now widespread, although they attract only a small proportion of those affected (Plass and Koch 2001; Grande *et al.* 2006). Their aim is to comfort, reassure, and discuss practical problems. A competently run support group will address participants' possible death and help them accept it. Humanistic–existential therapy (the two names are often bracketed and cover a variety of approaches, e.g. Spira 1997) goes further. It attempts to help patients find meaning in their lives by concentrating on the present sense of 'being' rather than on the past or the future. Attention is paid to such immediate issues as anxiety, awareness of mortality, lack of meaning, and the fear of taking responsibility for one's experience. This exploration may lead to a sense of authenticity that makes the approaching end of life more tolerable.

Spirituality adds an important further dimension: the idea that there is a transcendent, non-material order or intelligence that exists within and embraces us all, whether we know it or not. This order has been given many names: the Divine, God, the One, the Tao, the Source, the First Cause, Universal Intelligence, and so on. The great mystics, individuals who have realized their identity as part of this order, claim that our true selves are non-material and immortal. Psychospiritual therapy (Cunningham *et al.* 2001) attempts to help people experience this dimension of themselves (or, as might be said, the true Self behind the apparent separate self). With this understanding, it becomes clear why spirituality has so much to offer people with a terminal diagnosis: if we are more than just a body, then in some sense we are not bounded by birth and death. Religion may bring this type of solace, although it is important to distinguish spirituality, the quest for personal experience, from religions, which are institutionalized bodies of belief and practice based on an assumed underlying spiritual reality (Krippner 1995). When religious beliefs have simply been adopted uncritically, they may crumble under the threat of imminent death. In contrast, spiritual experience typically requires prolonged practice of skills and self-exploration and is more resistant to such threats.

## Research on clinical help in the spiritual domain

While spiritual concerns are recognized as important to many patients with cancer (Lin and Baur-Wu 2004; Villagomeza 2005), very little in the way of systematic spiritual help is usually offered, at least until the last stages of the disease (Miller *et al.* 2005; Chochinov 2006). There are very few descriptions in the literature of therapies with a strong spiritual component for ambulatory patients. Cole and Pargament (1999) reported on a brief group therapy program that had an explicitly spiritual aim. Breitbart *et al.* (2004) have described 'meaning-centred group psychotherapy', a brief therapy with a spiritual component. We (Cunningham 2005a) reported empirical results on the benefits to quality of life from a group psychospiritual program for 97 patients with varying types and stages of cancer.

The crucial importance of spirituality to people with life-threatening disease has always been understood by some mental health practitioners, as witnessed, for example, by the articles in a recent volume *Integrating Spirituality into*

*Treatment* (Miller 1999). Possible reasons for its non-inclusion in the usual treatment protocols for patients with cancer include:

- The materialistic focus of medical theory, which barely recognizes the importance of the mind, let alone the spirit, to health
- The general lack of interest in spirituality in Western culture (although there are many individual exceptions)
- The idea that spiritual care may be left to, or is the exclusive domain of, religious professionals
- A sense that there is little room for a proactive stance in promoting spiritual experience

## The 'Healing Journey' program

This program has been developed and conducted continuously for more than 25 years at a large metropolitan cancer treatment centre in Canada. Its main aim is to help patients and family members cope better with the disease, using psychological and spiritual ideas and practices. In recent years, as more intensive therapy aimed at inducing substantial change has been added to the program, we have investigated the possibility that it may prolong life in some participants. The Healing Journey has been adapted to meet the needs of patients presenting for this kind of help; thus, it depends on at least minimal willingness to practise basic coping skills, such as relaxation, and within a strongly multicultural community (Toronto) it has attracted mainly middle-class Caucasians (Cunningham *et al.* 1993). All aspects of the program have been subjected to research testing; thus, it is empirically, not ideologically, based.

Self-healing, the relief from suffering, is a process that can be learned. A teacher is generally required—the therapist is an educator. Like most learning processes, it is progressive, simple concepts and techniques being addressed before more complex ones. For the dedicated student, emotional and cognitive mastery of the crisis are achievable. We have found that it is most efficient to offer our courses in stepwise fashion, with a brief introductory class preceding increasingly demanding ones (Fig. 23.1). This allows patients to choose the extent and timing of their exposure to self-healing ideas and techniques. They can drop out at the end of any stage and resume the next at a later date if they wish. We work almost entirely with groups, both for reasons of economy and because the interactions between peers are extremely valuable in 'normalizing' the experience of individuals and providing emotional support. Participants are charged a small fee to reinforce the idea that this is something of value that they are doing for themselves.

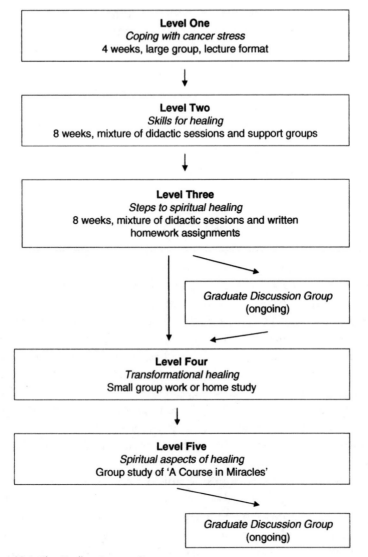

**Figure 23.1** The Healing Journey Program.

The techniques taught are drawn from various spiritual traditions and from psychological practice, a range of options being provided, so that individuals can select what 'works' for them. We begin with an introductory course comprising four weekly 1.5-hour interactive presentations by a leader to 40–80 participants in a small auditorium, repeated five times per year. The neutral title 'Coping with Cancer Stress' was chosen to attract as broad a spectrum of people as possible. The main concepts of self-healing are explained

(Cunningham 2000) and several basic self-help techniques are taught and practised: deep relaxation (two methods), thought monitoring and changing, visual imagery for healing, and defining goals. A workbook and CDs are supplied for home practice (available at www.healingjourney.ca). This course can also be offered to smaller numbers over six sessions, each including about an hour of supportive discussion. This basic course has been extensively researched using psychometric criteria and shown to lead to reliable improvements in quality of life, significantly greater than those achieved by support alone (Cunningham and Tocco 1989; Cunningham *et al.* 1999).

Because people's motivation varies so greatly, we have found that it is inefficient to increase the length of the basic course: many will drop out. Instead, we provide more advanced, short courses in a stepwise fashion. About one-half to two-thirds of first-level graduates proceed to a second-level class 'Skills for Healing' including eight weekly sessions. This develops the Level 1 techniques further—for example, participants now draw their 'healing imagery' in the class and have it critiqued—and we introduce journaling, consulting an 'Inner Healer', two methods of meditation, and the idea of undertaking a spiritual search. After an hour of didactic presentation and technique rehearsal, the class splits into smaller groups for supportive discussions. A workbook for home study is provided in this, as in all levels.

Level 3 for some years involved writing a 'life story' and presenting it to a small group (Cunningham and Edmonds 1996) but as our understanding of the potential of spiritual experience to affect health has grown, we have substituted an 8-week course 'Steps towards Spiritual Healing', in which we explore the way we create our experience through our inner monologue. This Level 3 course examines the pervasiveness of 'judgment' (emotion-laden reactivity to people and events), forgiveness, 'guilt' (self-judgment), projection, the need to feel 'special', and unconditional love (Cunningham 2002a). Further meditative techniques are taught and their practice encouraged. While standard psychological concepts are drawn upon, we also introduce a more 'spiritual' understanding of these topics. For example, forgiveness is seen not as a magnanimous overlooking of the transgressions of a less-aware person but as dropping our own internal judgmental reactions, a process aided by feeling connected to a spiritual source. We discuss the idea that there are many possible ways of thinking about a transcendent order or dimension, the important thing being to acquire one's own experience of it. This third-level course has been shown to improve quality of life significantly in 97 participants, over and above the improvements gained in the first two levels of the course (Cunningham 2005a).

These three initial levels, 20 weekly sessions in all, constitute our 'core program'. Graduates have been exposed to the main ideas and techniques commonly used in psychospiritual therapy and are encouraged to further their own healing by seeking out community institutions such as Buddhist centres, schools of personal growth, Sufi, Taoist, and yoga groups or by in-depth scriptural study at churches or synagogues. At the Healing Journey, we also provide twice-monthly 'drop in' discussion groups for them, at which we read and discuss the text of books by modern spiritual masters such as Eknath Easwaran and Eckhart Tolle.

Subsequent levels have a more explicitly spiritual orientation. Level 4, 'Transformational Healing,' is based directly on our published study (Cunningham and Watson 2004) of patients from our program with medically incurable cancers who have outlived their prognoses by between 4 and 14 years. Common features of these people were defined, by rigorous qualitative analysis, as 'authenticity', 'autonomy', and 'acceptance'. We have published some evidence to support the idea that learning to express these qualities might have the effect of inhibiting cancer growth (Cunningham *et al.* 2000a,b) and the course provides exercises and ideas designed to foster them. It is notable that they represent the opposite of the placatory, emotionally repressed 'Type C' adaptive style described as characteristic of many patients with cancer (Temoshok and Dreher 1992).

In Level 5, 'Spiritual Aspects of Healing', the aim is to develop a new way of viewing the world and one's place in it, consistent with the writings of the great mystics. Conventional materialism sees our experience of life as largely determined by outside events; introspective psychology can teach us that our experience is self-created; spiritual work introduces us to the still more radical idea that our material reality is also created by our thought—that thought is primary, the world secondary. Care is taken to avoid the naive assumption that we therefore may have 'caused our own cancers'; instead, it is pointed out that what we may have caused or created, collectively, is an idea of physical bodies in which cancer is possible. We have used various texts to explore these views but in the last 5 years have focused on *A Course in Miracles* (ACIM) (Foundation for Inner Peace 1996), which fits well into a psychologically based program for Western students. It is a profound, although difficult, text that invites readers to examine in depth how they have created their own sense of themselves, their 'egos', seen as separated from the Divine Ground. This course begins with 10 sessions of readings and exercises from ACIM and then continues as an ongoing, twice-monthly discussion group. We do not as yet have specific evidence to document the efficacy of this level of work, apart from some preliminary observations (still under analysis) that patients with metastatic disease who pursue the more intensive spiritual work live significantly longer than those who do not. Observationally, however, its effects on patients' life experience are often striking.

The Healing Journey appears to be the most developed program of its kind for patients with cancer, although it is possible that similar assistance is provided by individual therapists and non-orthodox organizations without being documented in the published literature. To recapitulate, the basic principles are: self-healing as something one learns; the use of a stepwise format and a wide range of techniques to accommodate individual preferences; and structuring the learning so that participants begin with basic coping skills, progress to changing habits of thought and only then to more explicitly spiritual work. These may seem rather obvious guidelines, but they do not appear to have influenced the psycho-oncology community. Instead, the norm in hospital settings is simply support groups for a small number of people. Where training in a coping skill such as meditation is offered, this is almost always restricted to a brief, single-level course. The practice of oncology is still a long way from routinely recommending the learning of coping skills as an integral part of the treatment of cancer, in spite of the fact that this is amply justified by the published literature on the benefits to quality of life.

## Planning further clinical research

Funding, publication space, and kudos currently tend to be awarded to studies carried out with strict experimental designs. Yet, at present, we have very little understanding of the factors promoting healing through mind and spirit—we need much more exploratory research to identify relevant variables and useful therapeutic approaches. While a randomized controlled trial might test whether, say, attendance at a meditation program enhances mean quality of life, it is an inappropriate means of examining the potential effects of spiritual study on lifespan in a situation where only a small proportion of patients make intensive use of a therapy. Nor will such a design facilitate analysis of the complex interacting variables that contribute to any result; observational data collection followed by qualitative analysis is much better suited to answering this kind of question (Cunningham 2002b; Cunningham 2005b). Shaping effective psychospiritual therapies is likely to be a gradual process of trial and adjustment. We need to draw on the writings of the mystics, as well as on clinical psychology and psychotherapeutic lore, and on our observations of many patients over time as they struggle with their healing. To explore the full potential of this kind of therapy to heal the physical body, we need to go far beyond what is customary in healthcare research, for example, by providing retreat settings where patients might devote themselves to healing work over a period of months; the costs would be amply justified if life were substantially prolonged. Therapists doing this kind of work obviously need their own spiritual experience, yet sufficient objectivity to avoid imposing their own ideologies on patients.

Spirituality has been 'coming out of the closet' in recent years as a legitimate subject for healthcare research. While this is very encouraging, we believe it is important in the cancer field, to go beyond the usual descriptive studies and explore interventions that may affect both the experience and the life spans of motivated individuals.

## Patients' statements about the benefits of psychospiritual therapy

In previous publications (Cunningham *et al.* 2001; Cunningham 2002a; Cunningham 2005a), we presented some comments of patients from our Level 3 course. For this chapter, we asked the members of the advanced *Course in Miracles* discussion group (all with 'incurable' diagnoses) to write something about their experience under the headings shown below.

### How has focusing on spiritual matters helped you cope with your cancer?

(NU): Developing a spiritual practice has provided me a ready 'refuge'. When my cancer diagnosis begins to become frightening or overwhelming, I can usually return to a place of calm fairly quickly through meditation or prayer.

(NE): Focusing on spiritual matters has given me guidance and support to face my fears and anxieties of the unknown. The spiritual path is a strength within me.

(TB): Somehow, the cancer itself became less important when I started focusing on spiritual matters. I still worry and there is still fear when I think about cancer or dying, but these feelings have become more manageable, and I no longer want to run away from them. At the same time, they seem to be less intense. The cancer is in my body, but I know I am not only my body.

### How has it affected your quality of life, i.e., your moods, thoughts, relationships?

(NU): It has greatly affected my quality of life. I am much more tolerant, much less a victim of my emotions. I am more quiet in my relationships, less demanding. I am less moody. I have a long, long ways to go yet, but I am very happy with what I have gained thus far.

(TX): The Healing Journey group has been fundamentally important in keeping me focused on appreciation, love and gratitude, and after seven years these have become habits. I do not suffer from dark thoughts as a rule, but when I do, I have tools to reframe, and I know what it means to feel peaceful and calm, and I am anxious to return to that state. In the same way, a spiritual lens gives me ways of letting go of my judgments about the countless ways in which my world is imperfect.

## What specific mental or spiritual techniques do you find most useful?

(NE): Daily meditation and reflection lets me experience my wholeness. I was diagnosed with cancer so I focus on the source of light which is what the Healing Journey is for me.

(TX): I listen to tapes or CDs of spiritual thinkers in the car, and at night when I have trouble sleeping—which is most nights. By now I have a rather extensive collection of Tolle, Pema Chodron, Levine, Thich Naht Hanh and Krishnamurti and these have become familiar and wonderful supports.

(DE): The spiritual techniques of meditation, spiritual readings, living in the now, yoga are all so interrelated that I cannot separate one from the other. I am truly at my best when I practise all of these on a regular basis.

## Has this work changed how you view your cancer and your mortality? Has it helped you see the purpose or meaning of your life differently?

(TB): This work has made me think about the purpose and the meaning of my life, which I hadn't done much before my diagnosis. I believe the purpose of my life is to understand my true nature and that I am part of the Divine.

(TX): It is not an exaggeration to say that focusing on spiritual matters has fundamentally shifted my view of the world, my work, my family and myself. I think this is what is often referred to as the *gift* of cancer ... The spiritual journey has reminded me of what I truly value and has inspired gratitude for the world I experience. In this 'revised' worldview, cancer is a blip, not the main focus, and I have come to understand healing as including myself and my relationships.

(ZM): Through my cancer experiences, through my work on spiritual healing, I faced the question 'What is the purpose of my life?' I learned it is not about materialism, it is not about me as a stand alone individual. It is about something much bigger. I am part of infinity, a part of God ... This new approach has given me a sense of peace and joy and a new outlook on my relations with others, for which I am grateful. I am grateful for every day.

(TH) I am not as fearful about physical death ... I believe that the physical body really wants to survive. I know that the spiritual being WILL. I have seen that physical death can be a very peaceful passing or filled with anger and distress. That has a lot to do with how life is lived.

### Have you had any unusual experiences that you would describe as 'spiritual'?

(NU) Absolutely. I have had several instances of being stopped in my tracks. It's often at odd times—unloading the groceries from my car, walking across the bridge on my way home, sitting on the bus. I become unable/unwilling to move, flooded with light, overwhelmed with joy and peace (it seems odd to be overwhelmed by such gentle feelings, but I don't know how else to describe it). These experiences last for 5–30 minutes. Also, when I meditate, at times I lose all sense of my physical body—I can't tell where it starts or stops, and I cannot feel the ground; it is as if I am floating.

(TX) My first reaction to this is that everything is spiritual—so that gratitude that comes in waves, or appreciation for the natural world, or people who touch my life are spiritual experiences. I have had incredible peace while meditating, and while just being still, and I think of this as spiritual—but not unusual. I envision healing white light—but it is not a spontaneous vision.

## Conclusion

Healing, which in its broadest sense is the relief from suffering, depends ultimately on resolving questions such as 'Why did this happen to me?' and 'Can I fit my illness, and hence my life as a whole, into some larger framework?' As shown by some of the preceding quotes, life-threatening illness can be seen as a call to investigate meaning in life. The likelihood of premature death only makes more urgent what spiritual masters have for millennia been describing as the main task of our lives. Of course, relatively few patients see it this way at first but with assistance, many are able to do so. As evidence accumulates on the benefits of a more holistic approach to serious illness, this approach may come to displace the prevailing current view of disease as a purely physical malfunction in the body machine and lead to more sophisticated therapy involving all dimensions of the patient.

## References

Breitbart, W., Gibson, C., Poppito, S. R. & Berg, A. 2004, Psychotherapeutic interventions at the end of life: a focus on meaning and spirituality, *Canadian Journal of Psychiatry*, vol. 49, no. 6, pp. 366–72.

Bultz, B. D. & Carlson, L. E. 2006, Emotional distress: the sixth vital sign - future directions in cancer care, *Psycho-oncology*, vol. 15, no. 2, pp. 93–5.

Chochinov, H. M. 2006, Dying, dignity and new horizons in palliative end-of-life care, *CA: Cancer Journal for Clinicians*, vol. 56, pp. 84–103.

Cole, B. & Pargament, K. 1999, Recreating your life: a spiritual/psychotherapeutic intervention for patients diagnosed with cancer, *Psycho-oncology*, vol. 8, pp. 395–407.

Cunningham, A. J. 2000, *The Healing Journey.* Key Porter Books. Toronto.

Cunningham, A. J. 2002*a*, *Bringing Spirituality into Your Healing Journey.* Key Porter Books, Toronto.

Cunningham, A. J. 2002*b*, Group psychological therapy: an integral part of care for cancer patients, *Integrative Cancer Therapies,* vol. **1**, no. 1, pp. 67–75.

Cunningham, A. J. 2005*a*, Integrating spirituality into a group psychological therapy program for cancer patients, *Integrative Cancer Therapies,* vol. **4**, no. 2, pp. 178–86.

Cunningham, A. J. 2005*b*, *Can the mind heal cancer?* A. J. Cunningham, Toronto.

Cunningham, A. J. & Edmonds, C. V. I. 1996, Adjuvant group psychological therapy for cancer patients: a point of view and discussion of the hierarchy of options, *International Journal of Psychiatry in Medicine,* vol. **26**, no. 1, pp. 51–82.

Cunningham, A. J. & Tocco, E. K. 1989, A randomized trial of group psychoeducational therapy for cancer patients, *Patient Education and Counseling,* vol. **14**, pp. 101–14.

Cunningham, A. J. & Watson, K. 2004, How psychological therapy may prolong survival in cancer patients: new evidence and a simple theory, *Integrative Cancer Therapies,* vol. **3**, pp. 214–29.

Cunningham, A. J., Edmonds, C. V. I. & Williams, D. 1999, Delivering a very brief psychoeducational program to cancer patients and their families in a large group format, *Psycho-oncology,* vol. **8**, pp. 177–82.

Cunningham, A. J., Edmonds, C. V. I., Phillips, C., Soots, K. I., Hedley, D., Lockwood, G. A. 2000*a*, A prospective longitudinal study of the relationship of psychological work to duration of survival in patients with metastatic cancer, *Psycho-oncology,* vol. **9**, pp. 323–39.

Cunningham, A. J., Phillips, C., Lockwood, G. A., Hedley, D. W. & Edmonds, C. V. I. 2000*b*, Do psychological self-regulation strategies prolong survival in patients with metastatic cancer? A prospective longitudinal study, *Advances in Mind Body Medicine,* vol. **16**, no. 4, 239–316.

Cunningham, A. J., Lockwood, G. A. & Edmonds, C. V. I. 1993, Which cancer patients benefit most from a brief, group, coping skills program?, *International Journal of Psychiatry in Medicine,* vol. **23**, no. 4, pp. 383–98.

Cunningham, A. J., Stephen, J., Phillips, C. & Watson, K. 2001, Psychospiritual therapy. In *Integrated Cancer Care: Holistic, Complementary and Creative Approaches,* pp. 173–86, (ed) J. Barraclough, Oxford University Press, Oxford.

Foundation for Inner Peace 1996, *A Course in Miracles.* Penguin Books, New York.

Grande, G. E., Myers, L. B. & Sutter, S. R. 2006, How do patients who participate in support groups differ from those who do not?, *Psycho-oncology,* vol. **15**, pp. 321–34.

Krippner, S. 1995, A cross-cultural comparison of four healing models, *Alternative Therapies,* vol. **1**, pp. 21–9.

Lin, H. R. & Baur-Wu, S. M. 2004, Psycho-spiritual well-being in patients with advanced cancer: an integrative review of the literature, *Journal of Advanced Nursing,* vol. **44**, no. 1, pp. 69–80.

Miller, D. K., Chibnall, J. T., Videen, S. D. & Duckro, P. N. 2005, Supportive affective group experience for persons with life threatening illness: reducing spiritual, psychological and death related distress in dying patients, *Journal of Palliative Medicine,* vol. **8**, no. 2, pp. 333–43.

Miller, W. R. 1999, *Integrating spirituality into treatment.* American Psychological Association, Washington DC.

Plass, A. & Koch, U. 2001, Participation of oncological outpatients in psychosocial support, *Psycho-oncology*, vol. **10**, pp. 511–20.

Ryan, H., Schofields, P., Cockburn, J. *et al.* 2005, How to recognize and manage psychological distress in cancer patients, *European Journal of Cancer Care*, vol. **14**, pp. 7–15.

Spira, J. L. 1997, *Group Therapy for Medically Ill Patients*. Guilford Press, New York.

Temoshok, L. & Dreher, H. 1992, *The Type C Connection: The Behavioral Links to Cancer and Your Health*. Random House, New York.

Vachon, M. 2006, Psychosocial distress and coping after cancer treatment, *American Journal of Nursing*, vol. **106**, no. 3, pp. 26–31.

Villagomeza, L. R. 2005, Spiritual distress in adult cancer patients: toward conceptual clarity, *Holistic Nursing Practice*, Nov–Dec, pp. 285–94.

# Index